handling

MR. HYDE

handling
MR. HYDE

questions and answers about
manic depression

Stanley A. Katz M.D., Ph.D.
Ira M. Katz Ph.D.

Handling Mr. Hyde, Questions and Answers About
Manic Depression
Stanley A. Katz, MD, PhD
Ira M. Katz, PhD

Cover Design and Interior Typography: Anna
McBrayer

ISBN: 1-887617-18-3

For our mother
Bernice M. Katz, Ph.D.

table of contents

preface

Imagine an illness that strikes at the beginning of the prime of life, robbing an individual of his insight and personality to such an extent that he might lose his career, wealth, friends, family and even his life. This is the nature of manic depression (bipolar disorder). The most problematic symptom that patients, their families and friends must deal with is the loss of personality. Because of this loss the patient loses insight, so much so that for the intents and purposes of assistance, the person who inhabited the body is no longer present. But a different person, one who believes all is well, now inhabits the body. Thus the disease, the real enemy, seems to be one and the same with the person who needs help.

Therefore, this disease might best be understood through the popular story *The Strange*

Case of Dr. Jekyll and Mr. Hyde by Robert Louis Stevenson. In that story Dr. Jekyll takes a potion that transforms his body and mind into Mr. Hyde. Thus, the friends of Jekyll cannot reason with him when he is Hyde. This story, although it has major differences from manic depression that we will describe, can give the reader an understanding of the loss of personality due to manic depression. We have chosen to title this book *Handling Mr. Hyde* for two primary reasons. First, just as Jekyll had to rectify the damage induced by Hyde, the patient when healthy must deal with the overwhelming problems incurred by his mania. Second, because it is imperative for those involved with the care of someone stricken with this disorder to realize that the person they are trying to help is not the one who disdains assistance. This crucial lesson is very often lost on the families of those who suffer from manic depression. Thus, this book is intended to assist people afflicted with manic depression by educating patients and their loved ones about the many ramifications involved with the control of this complicated illness, which extend well beyond medicine into virtually every aspect of life.

Our writing stems from our direct experience with the disease for more than a decade:

Stan suffering from the illness and his brother Ira attempting to help him. Needless to say we have had exposure to numerous psychiatrists and medications as well as other ancillary therapies. We have listened to academic seminars and presentations from some of the experts in the field, studied the literature, and attended countless hours in support groups. There have been admissions to over 10 hospitals including private, university and state institutions. These hospitalizations have been both voluntary and involuntary, at times with police involvement. On one occasion Stan was taken to jail. We have also dealt with the courts on several occasions. The illness has resulted in Stan being dismissed from jobs five times and losing all of his savings and personal possessions. We have applied for Social Security and other benefits, shopped for health insurance and battled financial devastation.

Moreover, we bring a unique perspective to this topic because of our backgrounds. Stan is a physician who has had residency training in psychiatry, internal medicine and neurology. In addition both of us have doctorate degrees (Stan in physiology, Ira in mechanical engineering) providing advanced scientific knowledge. Perhaps there is no other person with the training and firsthand knowledge that Stan brings to this discussion. We considered writing an academic text. But we feel this book, directed at those people whose lives are touched by manic depression every day, would be much more helpful. Furthermore, beyond scientific knowledge, we have a fresh approach into the workings of society in general that will help the reader understand why mental illness is so difficult to treat.

There have been celebrities who have written books or publicly discussed their manic depression. For example, the experiences of Patty Duke, Kristy McNichol, Brian Wilson, Margot Kidder, Connie Francis and Vivien Leigh have been recounted in the popular media. Perhaps the most relevant to this work is Kay Redfield Jamison, who has written widely about manic depression based on her experience as a patient and psychologist. All of these efforts in some sense are helpful to patients and families. We, however, write from the experience of ordinary citizens, albeit with extraordinary academic qualifications, who explain the fundamental elements of the disease itself and how it must be dealt with. For example, negotiating with the police or an employer is different for us than it is for a celebrity. The details of these kinds of experiences are also seldom addressed in the existing accounts. For these reasons we think this book will be more relevant for most people.

The book is made up of eight chapters. Four of the chapters are essays that cover a specific topic in depth. But as the subtitle indicates, the core of the book is the other four chapters that consist of questions and answers about manic depression. When we say "answers" we do not mean to infer that appropriate action can be prescribed on every occasion. In many instances there is no ultimate solution available; one can only cope with the situation by realizing that this is a chronic, incurable illness. Once this fact is accepted, mitigating circumstances should be recognized and acted upon in a positive manner when the opportunity arises. Stan, Ira or both provide the answers to each question. Thus, this format allows for at least three voices: that of the patient, who is also able to provide the viewpoint of the physician, and the family, as necessary. For example, we both offer unique perspectives on our individual experiences during Stan's manic episodes, our interactions with psychiatrists, the status of mental hospitals and numerous others. Thus, we provide detailed descriptions of how to recognize and deal with problems using examples from our own experience. We hope this format will allow readers to jump into the body of the book at any point to meet their particular needs and to feel that they are part of a conversation. However, the book is also designed to be read straight through.

The question-and-answer format has evolved from the hours of conversation we have had with friends and acquaintances relating our experiences. We have seen estimates that as many as 2.5 million people suffer from this disease in the United States. The disease also affects many more millions of family members and friends. Yet very few people admit to this problem in themselves or even in their families for several reasons, which will be explored in detail. For instance, in most settings manic depression is only mentioned in the form of amusement or ridicule about who should be taking his lithium. There is a significant stigma associated with those affected by manic depression and other mental illnesses. Very few people have an understanding or appreciation of what the disease actually entails. A major goal of this work is to provide this education.

Chapter 1 is a description by Ira of the series of events that occurred as a result of Stan's manic episode in 1994 that resulted in Stan travelling to Hawaii from his home in Kentucky. This chapter straightforwardly relates the human toll exacted by the disease on virtually all aspects of life of the patient and the family.

Chapter 2 is the first of the question-and-answer chapters. It consists of questions that directly concern how the physiological nature of the illness causes behavioral symptoms. This very complex topic is usually the first hurdle of understanding that those affected by the disease must overcome. We emphasize that this is an organic illness. Then we describe the textbook definition that psychiatrists employ in arriving at the diagnosis. The roles of genetic and environmental factors in causing the illness are examined. Last we describe how the illness is manifested, with Stan providing details of his own manic episodes and depressions.

Chapter 3 is Stan's essay on the complicated subject of the pharmacology of manic depression, that includes a fundamental discussion of the structure and function of the brain and its building blocks, the nerve cells. The description of the pertinent biochemical processes thought to be involved in this disease will illuminate how and why particular medications are initiated, emphasizing that they absolutely do not cure the illness.

If the illness has been identified, how is it treated? This is the central question of Chapter 4. The primary topics of importance are the care provided by psychiatrists and hospitals, and a recap of the role of medications. Intertwined in this chapter we discuss the pivotal role that the family must maintain in the chronic care of this illness that often supercedes any other approach to treatment.

Chapter 5 is an essay on free will that addresses the issue of whether or not a person suffering from manic depression is responsible for his actions. It is fundamental that families understand this issue if they are to help a loved one.

Chapter 6 consists of questions related to personal relationships and day-to-day issues involved in coping with the disease. Of primary importance is the effect of the illness on relationships, because it is terribly difficult for a patient to control the treatment and ramifications of manic depression alone.

Chapter 7 is an essay on bureaucracy that explains how societal constraints make it more difficult to assist the mentally ill. This concerns not just government workers, but police, the justice system and businesses that are also bureaucratic in nature.

Chapter 8 broadens the scope of Chapters 6 and 7 to the wider society. How does society deal with manic depression? How do businesses, government services, the judicial system, etc., interact with people with manic depression? How do those interactions exacerbate the devastation to career and finances that this illness can cause?

An Epilogue follows, addressing the current state of Stan's health and care.

We hope that this book might be of help to those who are affected by other mental illnesses, especially the related diseases clinical depression and schizophrenia. The most profound similarity is the loss of personality that makes caring for another so difficult, in other words, the appearance of Mr. Hyde.

Finally, we would like to thank the many people who have read the manuscript, especially M. McDevitt, Ph.D. and E. Starr, Ph.D.

Stanley A. Katz, M.D., Ph.D.
Ira M. Katz, Ph.D.
July 2001

chronology of events
related to the illness

April 1960–Born, Chicago, IL

December 1981– Graduates first in class, electrical engineering, Clemson University

June 1982–Enters M.D./Ph.D. program, Medical University of South Carolina at Charleston

October 1986–First manic (psychotic) episode, hospitalization, subdued with Haldol, starts treatment with lithium

May 1989–Completes M.D./Ph.D.

July 1989–Begins internship, U.N.C.–Chapel Hill

June 1990–Completes internship

August 1990–Begins neurology residency, U.N.C.-Chapel Hill

October 1990–Brief manic episode, no hospitalization

February 1991–Manic episode, discards possessions, hospitalization at Durham County General for two weeks

March 1991–Released while still manic, hospitalized at Duke University Hospital, transferred after first being admitted to U.N.C. hospital to protect reputation

April 1991–Insurance exhausted, transferred to State Mental Hospital, Butner, NC, begins using Tegretol with lithium

May 1991–Released from hospital and residency position, U.N.C.

January 1992–Begins neurology residency, Vanderbilt University, Nashville, TN

April 1992–Manic episode, discards possessions, hospitalization, begins low dose of Haldol in addition to Tegretol and lithium

October 1992–Released from residency position, Vanderbilt University

July 1993–Begins neurology residency, University of Kentucky, Lexington, KY

March 1994–Not reappointed to residency position, University of Kentucky

October 1994–Manic episode, discards possessions, travels to Hawaii, hospitalization, discharged on Haldol, Tegretol and lithium

January 1995–Begins general medical practice, Bay Springs, MS

January 1995–Manic episode, hospitalization, ineffective treatment with Haldol, Tegretol and lithium

April 1995–Moves to San Antonio with mother to be near Ira, begins treatment with valproic acid monotherapy

September 1995–Begins psychiatry residency, University of Texas Health Science Center at San Antonio

November 1995–Profiled for Abbot Laboratories, producer of valproic acid, stock report

February 1996–Manic episode, dismissed from residency position, University of Texas Health Science Center at San Antonio

May 1996–Arrested in Nashville, TN

April 1998–Siezed by police in Maryland and hospitalized, begins Depakote and low dose of antipsychotic olanzapine

July 1998–Moves to Florida to be near brother Mike

July 1999–Receives disability assistance for the first time

chapter one:
my trip to Hawaii or Stan's latest episode

This narrative was written to describe to friends my experiences in helping Stan deal with a major manic episode. Many of the problematic situations with police, social workers, and businesspeople discussed here are typical of what I have encountered over the years. The disruptive force of a manic episode on the family is also apparent in this account. This essay, originally written as an e-mail, is a written version of my oral description of the events; therefore, it came about that I wrote it without breaking the sections into paragraphs.

Kentucky

This summer Stan went through the difficult experience of being fired from his neurology residency position at the University of Kentucky. The firing was unfair but after some thought of suing, we decided it was best to just move on. He came down to Texas (where I was living) to visit and recover his mental stability. We discussed his career plans. I suggested he look for a small practice where he could treat patients, not be on call and be away from the (expletive deleted) doctors who make up academic medicine in this country. Several weeks later he received an offer and decided to accept a position in a small town in Mississippi. It was just what I had in mind for him. A 4-1/2-day work week, virtually no call (not being at work but available in emergency situations) and a community that was looking forward to welcoming him. The guaranteed $125,000-a-year salary was not bad either. About six weeks ago Stan went down to Mississippi to get his license and make other arrangements for his move. Upon his return to Lexington we talked. He had bought a house down there on the spur of the moment. By all indications this was a good buy, but Stan seemed a bit too excited. He kept saying he bought the house for me. The next day we talked again and other signs of mania were creeping into his thoughts. My mother and other brother also noticed these signs. I knew Stan was seeing his psychiatrist that day; he said he was still taking his medication, but we were very concerned. I tried to call his psychiatrist for three days without success. Finally on Friday I contacted him. The psychiatrist had heard from Stan's apartment manager that he was acting strange. I called Stan and told him to go to the doctor's. He agreed. I called the doctor again to check if the had taken Stan to the hospital. Well, someone had seen Stan in the building but now they could not find him. The doctor was also leaving for the weekend. I knew then that I needed to go to Lexington to get Stan in the hospital. I had planned to leave that day for Gainesville to attend the Auburn-Florida football game. I called my friends from the airport telling them that I could not attend. I arrived in Lexington at about 10 PM Friday. No rental cars were available because the races were on at Keenland (horse racing), University of Kentucky had midnight madness basketball and there was a big gun show in town. So I took a cab to Stan's apartment. He was not there and I could see through the window that he had thrown out his possessions once again. My next thought was to get a room for the night. The same cabby (who had a B.A. in English, was a C.P.A., and was now driving cabs and training thoroughbreds) took me to a couple of motels that were full. I was told that all the rooms in Lexington were full for that night. I had the cab take me to the police station. I filed a missing-person report and tried to get a magistrate's order to have the police help me get him to the hospital if required. That turned out to be a major bureaucratic nightmare on a Friday night. I went back to the police station and asked if they had any ideas where I could stay that night. The detective said that the Kimball House would have rooms. "It is not much to look at, but the rooms are clean." I walked the few blocks to the place and found an old-style boarding house. The lady at the desk looked about 70 years old and was wearing a Victorian, starched, high-collared shirt. The room had a small black-and-white TV that only picked up three UHF channels. I was ready for a beer at that point. But she mentioned that they lock the doors after 12. There was a buzzer you could press to be let in. I asked who would let me in. She said "me or my husband." Well I couldn't wake the old folks up so I watched U.K. midnight madness on my little B&W. The next day I walked back to the police station: no word on Stan. I then caught a cab to Stan's apartment. They let me in but it was cleaned out, except for the furniture. I decided to watch the game I was supposed to attend because there was nothing else to be done. It was a great game but the Gators lost on a last-second touchdown. Nothing was going right. My Mom kept calling, even though I had nothing new to report, because she had become irrational. I went back to San Antonio the next day. As I came in the door my phone was ringing. It was my Mom's neighbor. My Mom was drinking gin and saying she wanted to commit suicide. What a weekend!

Hawaii

The next few days I waited to see if Stan would show up in Kentucky from my home in Texas. The Lexington police found his car at the airport. He left it unlocked with the keys inside. Through his credit card company I found out that he had purchased jewelry (an engagement ring) and stayed at the Lexington Hilton the Friday night I was at the Kimball House. I then learned he purchased two tickets to Hawaii and two were used. I still do not know about that second ticket (it turns out it was not used). Now I knew he was in Hawaii but not where. Finally he was tracked down by the Lexington police to the Princeville Hotel on Kauai. I made contact with the Kauai police and mental health authorities. They found Stan but they would not admit him to the hospital involuntarily. Once again I knew that if I did not find him and get him in the hospital nobody would. That night some friends from my academic department had a dinner party. I finally went home about 10. My $1600 flight the next morning was at 6:00 so I was up by 4:00. The flight went from San Antonio to Dallas to Los Angeles to Maui to Honolulu to Lihue on Kauai. When I arrived in Lihue I planned on catching a cab to the hotel, looking for Stan, and then getting him to the hospital. When I learned the cab fair was $62 I decided to check with the hotel if they had a shuttle. No shuttle was available and even more of a problem was that Stan had checked out that morning. I took a cab to the police station once again. This time the cabby was a pain. It was less than two miles to the station and the fare was $5.25. I had a $20 bill to pay him. He had no change. I would take $10 as change but he had nothing. Then he told me the meter was still running. There was nobody I could talk to at the station to get change. Finally I told him to take me to get some change. We stopped at a liquor store where they would not give me change unless I purchased something (a pack of gum). When we got back to the station the fare was now $6.25. I paid him the exact amount. The Kauai police are definitely not Hawaii-5-0. I asked if they would check the airlines to see if he had left the island. "No, I do not want to lose my job." Can I talk to somebody to give you authority, like a magistrate or a judge? "It is the weekend and nobody ever calls the judge on the weekend." I said I would call and he simply gave me a phone book. Of course the office was closed on the weekend and I didn't know the name of the judge. I gave up looking for Stan for the day, except for the minimal task of filling out a missing-person report. They asked where I was staying on the island. I replied, "I don't know, I just got here from Texas." One of them mentioned a hotel on the beach, another told me about the Tip Top Motel around the corner. I didn't feel like taking another cab that night so I headed for the Tip Top. The office was closed when I arrived at about 9 PM. There was a little bar, called Charley and Chrissy's Place, located in the same building so I checked to see if I could get a room from there. It was a small place with a Hawaiian woman bartending and a man drinking a beer. I asked for a Budweiser and inquired about a room. The bartender got a quarter and made a phone call from the pay phone on the wall. About 20 minutes later another woman arrived with her hair in curlers. This was Chrissy. I got hooked up with a room, this time with a new cable TV system. The new system didn't work so I decided to have another beer. I mentioned that my TV didn't work. Shortly thereafter a little Chinese fellow, smoking a cigarette, wearing no shirt, came into the bar and inquired about my malfunctioning TV. This was Charley. We walked over to my room to check it out. While puffing away, he attempted to get the TV to work but failed, so we walked to the room next door where the TV did work. I found out that Charley and Chrissy live in a room at the motel (they are small rooms) and run the bar. They will also check people into the motel if the office is closed. At the close of the day Saturday my plan was to get authorization for Stan to be committed on Monday, if he was still on the island, and leave on the red-eye to arrive back in San Antonio for my class on Tuesday. My flight was originally scheduled for Tuesday so I changed it that night. My first few hours in Kauai were very frustrating so I was anxious to leave. Sunday morning I walked over to the police station. I did not expect anything new but this seemed to me as good a starting place as any other. The officer on duty was much more cooperative than the officers from the night before. After I described the situation to him, he attempted to retrieve the missing-person report I had filed the day before. There was no report in the files. He asked when I had filed my report. After I explained to him my previous visit, he instructed me never to do anything with the police between 2:00 and 11:00 because that shift always screws up! Fine, I thought to myself, I would try and check things out myself. I called a cab company that services the Princeville Hotel, but they could give me no information. I then walked over to the airport. I was still loath to use a cab. I told my story to both Aloha and Hawaiian Airlines, the two carriers who work the inter-island routes. One of the supervisors checked the records for me: no Stan. The other said he would check if a police officer were there. Of course the police said they had no authority. There was nothing more I could do for Stan until offices opened the next day so I decided to play golf. I saw a brochure at the airport for a course and went there by cab. Fifteen miles and $35 later I was at the Kiahuna Golf Club. The $45 green fee and cart rental were not too bad, but I also needed clubs, balls, and a glove, which brought the total to $100. The course was OK but I really wanted to hit a ball into the Pacific and this course was not on the ocean. There were some hotels nearby so I decided to walk on over to see if I could eat lunch looking over the ocean. I was very disappointed because most of the establishments along the beach were closed due to damage incurred by Hurricane Iniki two years previous. As nothing was open I decided to return to Lihue. I did not want to call a cab; I thought I might have to pay double the fare to have it come out and take me back to Lihue. $135 was already enough for this round of golf. I had nothing better to do and I was in Hawaii, so I started walking with my thumb extended. After a mile or so I was picked up. This ride got me to a little town that was still 10 miles from the Tip Top. But there was a restaurant-bar. I stopped in for a couple of cold ones and a bowl of chili. Everyone at the bar was big with long hair, and tattoos. I peered out the window and noticed the row of Harley motorcycles for the first time. After being refreshed with my libations I hit the road again. I was walking past sugar cane fields, which were being harvested. It was interesting, but the sickly-sweet odor was not pleasant. Eventually another chap picked me up. He took me almost all the way back into Lihue. I still wanted to eat on the ocean so I kept on walking to find the locals' beach. I relaxed while reading, drinking a beer, eating, and watching the waves roll in and the little mice which were running up to my table. It was then another two to three miles walk back to the Tip Top, where I stopped in at Charley and Chrissy's room to pay for another night. Monday morning I made contact with the mental health authorities. The social worker was a very nice person, but not very effective, and very much a bureaucrat. He would not do a thing until it was cleared by his boss, a psychiatrist. I explained the situation to this doctor and explained what I wanted done. From my previous experiences with Stan's illness I had come to understand the law. His first words to me were "Are you an attorney?" He basically agreed with what I said and told the social worker to help me find him. It turns out that the hotel had given some information to the mental health people about Stan's whereabouts. He had apparently rented a condominium close to the hotel. The drive out to Princeville from Lihue took about 30 minutes. It was a nice drive and it gave me the opportunity to see more of the island. The social worker was a pleasant fellow but inept. We found the condo Stan had rented. The door was wide open but nobody was there. I walked in to investigate; John, the social worker, wouldn't. It was definitely Stan's place. I found the engagement ring. He had also bought a couple of new tennis rackets. We checked with the office staff. The manager knew nothing except that the unit was rented out by Mimsy Bouret and owned by her husband, Pierre. We decided to go down the road to the hotel Stan had been at to see if we could get any leads there before checking with the Bouret's. The Princeville Hotel is the nicest hotel I have ever been in. It is plush, with large fountains in the lobby. It is situated on Manalai Bay. This is the location where the movie *South Pacific* was filmed. There are two great golf courses there. The room rate is about $300/night. As we walked through the lobby I thought this place was a cut above the Tip Top. The staff remembered Stan. We asked that they contact John if he was seen there again. We then went to see Mimsy. She was very nice, but quirky. Pierre appeared to be a West Coast beach bum who had been in the sun for 40 years. Upon introducing myself as Stan's brother Mimsy asked if there was a problem with the rental. I replied in the affirmative. Mimsy said, "I knew something like this would happen on a Monday." Stan was paying $2,000 a month for the gorgeous condo. He had taken a two-month lease and had already put down a $1,600 deposit. Pierre then walked in and said he had just seen Stan about 15 minutes ago in the same shopping center as the realty office. We were close. We drove around the area for about an hour, back to the condo and around again to the shopping center. I finally spotted him walking beside the road. He greeted me and was very cooperative. This has not always been the case in the past when Stan was manic. It took about three more hours of driving and interviews with doctors to finally get him into the psychiatric ward of the hospital. At one point the psychiatrist told me he would not have committed him except for the fact that I was present to explain the lack of reality in Stan's account of his stay in Hawaii. It was a great relief to finally have Stan in the hospital.

The Return

There was no chance of making my flight on Monday so I changed it back to Tuesday. I rented a car and headed back out to Princeville. My plan was to spend the night at Stan's fabulous condo, then in the morning get all his possessions in order, straighten things out with Mimsy and the bank, pick a up few things which he might need in the hospital, visit with him and his doctor and then catch the afternoon plane back to San Antonio. After arriving back at the condo I was intent on watching the sunset over the Pacific while drinking a beer. I wandered over to the hotel and watched one of the most spectacular sunsets I had ever seen with a cold Bud. There must have been a score of what looked like honeymoon couples taking pictures. I had a nice meal and settled in at the condo for the night. I was still maintaining Central Time throughout this trip so I awoke around 2:00 in the morning. I made several phone calls back east to my family, doctors, and future employers. At daybreak I was ready for the day. I had a few hours until Mimsy and the bank would be open so I decided to take a drive up the coast. The northeast coast of Kauai is a national park with no roads. The drive to the park is rural and scenic. I hiked up a trail several hundred yards. It was very steep and rocky, through dense tropical foliage, until there was a clear path to a cliff overlooking the ocean. There was a wonderful fresh breeze and the view was spectacular. But what made the view special was the tiny rain cloud that had drifted over the ocean from the center of the island. The mountains in the center of Kauai have the highest rainfall of any spot on earth. From this tiny misting cloud an intense rainbow appeared which joined the grey-white puff to the calm sea below. I was the only witness to this hopeful sign from above. I headed back to Princeville, stopping to have breakfast at a local joint decorated with surfing pictures. It would turn out that the large omelet and hash browns would be my only sustenance for far longer than I had anticipated. I first talked to Mimsy. Stan had thrown away the realtor's lock box and the keys to the condo. His lease also kept her from renting the place to another party. I suppose Stan was liable for the full $4,000 but hopefully he would be able to get some money back. Stan had also transferred much of his money to a bank in Hawaii. I talked to the manager about restoring the funds back to Kentucky. I did not have the authority at that time to return the funds, but this was not a problem as this was accomplished after our return. I then picked up several items from the store that could be of use to Stan in the hospital and started back to Lihue. Stan was in a good (manic) mood when I arrived. We had as positive a talk as is possible when he is in that state. Of greatest importance was his compliance with treatment in the hospital. I then sat down to have a chat with the doctor before heading to the airport. He suggested that I take Stan back home. It would save much hassle and money to take him now rather than later and Stan seemed cooperative with me. I dreaded the thought but had to agree. I told Stan; he was excited about taking an airplane trip with me. Oh boy! So I called Delta again to change my flight to Lexington and purchased a ticket for Stan. With the doctor assisting, I arranged a medical emergency fare that saved me several hundred dollars. Our itinerary took us from Lihue on Kauai to Honolulu via Aloha Airlines. From there we took Delta nonstop to Atlanta and then on to Lexington. I discussed with the doctor in Lexington the arrangements for Stan's hospital admittance. As one might imagine, my senses were keen to Stan's every movement. It turned out he was as cooperative as I could have hoped for. He did go to the bathroom often, and he spilled a Coke at the airport, and told me the wrong gate information, but I could think of many scenarios that are much worse. By the time we arrived in Lexington Wednesday morning I had not slept more than 15 minutes since waking up Tuesday. I had not eaten anything except a couple of bites of horrible plane food since my omelet. But I was so involved with what needed to be done that I was not tired or hungry. We were both dressed for the tropical Kauai climate. The temperature was 40°F in Lexington. I went to hail a cab but there were none available. I was so close to getting him to the hospital and now no cabs. This was very frustrating. I finally arranged for transportation to the hospital (but we were also stopped by a train) where Stan was admitted. I made a couple of local calls in Lexington to the police and Stan's apartment complex. Then it was on to the airport to purchase another ticket back to San Antonio through Atlanta. I arrived back home about 9 PM. I went by my school and the post office to sort through my mail and messages, then I returned home to sleep. The next day (Thursday) I explained to my classes what had happened to me and told them the revised schedule for their assignments. Then it was back to the airport. Several months ago I had made nonrefundable, unchangeable reservations to go to Knoxville for a wedding. So I went to Atlanta and on to Knoxville. I also had the same reservations for the following week for a second Knoxville wedding. I am tired of eating Delta turkey sandwich snacks.

Epilogue

As of this writing Stan is still in the hospital. Many of his delusions persist. I am confident he will come out of it eventually. I am not sure about his job in Mississippi. I suspect that sometime I will need to get him into the hospital again. Many people ask when I tell them this story if I get depressed in dealing with this situation (or "burden" as we tend to call family troubles these days). I do not. I only think of the task ahead in fulfilling my responsibility. I also realize that everyone has "burdens." I see the problems others must deal with around the world and I count my blessings that I do not live in Somalia or Rwanda. While in Hawaii I was reading *Uncle Tom's Cabin* by Harriet Beecher Stowe. How could I lament my situation compared to what the slaves endured? Even more relevant, I recognize how much more difficult it is for Stan. The point is that feeling sorry for yourself never helps the situation. So I recognize the good fortune I have had in my life and try to meet my responsibilities with good cheer.

chapter two:
what is manic depression?

---

1. What is manic depression?

Stan: Manic depression is a mental illness that is expressed as abnormalities in mood that can vary from the deep depths of an all-consuming, suicidal hopelessness to euphoric insanity. This disease is thus called bipolar disorder in the medical literature, in contrast to the mood disorder major depression, that is termed unipolar. Manic depression is an organic illness–the malfunctioning or diseased organ is the brain. This point must be emphatically emphasized, namely that it is a pathologic medical condition similar to cancer, heart disease or diabetes. Because the primary symptoms are of emotion, thought and behavior as opposed to physical symptoms related to other organ ailments, most people do not recognize this fact.

Bipolar illness strikes people of all races and social classes. It is seen in one percent of the population, with men and women equally afflicted. In contrast, the incidence of major depression (the unipolar disorder) is two times more common in females than males. The risk for symptoms in women for both disorders increases during the post-partum (after childbirth) period. Some people seem to have relapses only at certain times of the year, which is referred to as seasonal variation. The usual age of onset is in the early 20's but it can begin in adolescence or middle age. More recently, some researchers have come to believe that children may also develop symptoms.

Ira: To reemphasize what Stan has written, the most important point to understand is that manic depression is an organic disease. Just as the organs the heart, kidney, or gall bladder might not function properly, the organ called the brain can malfunction. This malfunction of the brain is expressed as a change in personality or mood. Of course, there are many valid, that is environmental, reasons for a change in mood. All of us have been depressed. For example, imagine a terrible event has occurred in your life, such as your parents being killed in an automobile accident. You would understandably feel sad, lethargic, lose your appetite-you may even think of suicide. All of these moods are somehow manifested in your brain chemistry. But what if your brain chemistry expressed this mood without the occurrence of a terrible event but due to a malfunction of your brain? This is major (or clinical) depression. The novelist William Styron has described his depression in the book *The Darkness Visible*. Because of his illness he believed his career was failing when it was at its height. Recognizing diseases such as depression and manic depression is complicated by the fact that both the organic chemical effects due to the illness and environmental chemical effects are always operating in tandem and cannot be isolated from one another.

2. How is manic depression diagnosed?

Stan: Following years of study, physicians have compiled a list of symptoms that categorize the illness. That is, the somewhat subjective observation of a patient's behavior is the only way to detect the illness. There is no objective blood test or imaging device available to assist in diagnosis or treatment. The defining criteria of behavior most widely employed today are listed in the American Psychiatric Association's Diagnostic and Statistical Manual of *Mental Disorders, Fourth Edition (DSM-IV)*. I will translate the medical definition of bipolar disorder as described in the *DSM-IV* into a form that I hope can be understood by non-specialists. I will also describe some of my personal experiences with the disease as they apply, so that the reader can gain insight into these symptoms that are frequently difficult to relate to or comprehend for the average person. The presence of a manic episode is what defines one as having manic depression. According to the *DSM-IV,* to be considered manic, one must experience a persistent, expansive or euphoric mood of at least one week in duration (or less time if severe enough to necessitate hospitalization). Mood refers to one's inner feelings or state of mind reflected in speech, appearance and behavior in general. Besides having an elevated mood, a person can also be considered to be having a manic episode if his mood is irritable or angry. In such a person a euphoric state will usually occur prior to the irritable state. This is especially true when the person in the elevated mood has his way or plans stifled. Sometimes there can be a rapid alternation between the two states.

The *DSM-IV* lists seven symptoms that may occur during this period of mood disturbance. Three of the seven are required for the "objective" diagnosis of a manic state. If the mood is irritable, four of these are required. I have placed objective in quotes because these are actually quite subjective, and often are not witnessed by others, including the psychiatrist. In fact, psychiatrists can rarely directly observe many of the symptoms the patient has suffered during the episode, because the symptoms are not usually all expressed at any particular time. Additionally, symptoms may be concealed by the patient to avoid hospitalization. Information from the family is critical to determine the previous level of functioning of the patient. Furthermore, the family can reveal the timeline of the symptoms. This will have a significant impact on the ability to establish the diagnosis. In the process of determining the diagnosis it is often difficult to categorize a particular behavior as one distinct symptom, making the count towards diagnosis uncertain. Furthermore, knowl-edge of the family history of mental illness should inform the diagnosis due to the strong genetic predisposition to the disease. The seven symptoms are considered below.

(1) Bipolar patients may demonstrate an increase in self-esteem or expansiveness by expressing thoughts that they are more beau-tiful or intelligent than in the past, and expressing these thoughts in numerous social settings. Furthermore, they may be grandiose to the extent of believing they have the greatest talent of anyone in the world at some endeavor (such as in singing, sports, acting, politics, etc.). It should be readily obvious that this grandiosity could contribute toward producing a euphoric state. An engineer at a support group I attended related that during a manic episode he thought he had discovered a new concept for flight. He put much of this on paper, but when he recovered he realized his design was totally ridiculous.

My mania began with confidence increased to the point of ignoring personal problems, and euphoria associated with an incessant desire to listen to loud rock music.

From that point I started to believe my research work would be highly significant in the annals of medicine. This grandiosity then escalated to my believing that I was the greatest tennis player in the world, and that I would be the next president of the United States. Finally, my thinking culminated with my belief that I was God. Bear in mind that with some episodes there was no progression, but an almost instantaneous belief that I was God. Given my knowledge of the illness and not wanting to be considered sick and placed in the hospital, I sometimes answered questions on this topic in an evasive manner. When a psychiatrist asked me if I "thought" I would be president of the United States or if I "thought" I was God, I answered "no." This was truthful for I "knew" I would be president and I "knew" I was God. Of course when not manic I would not mince words and would desire medical care. To sum up, when manic, a patient has a tremendous shift in personality-this is the presence of Mr. Hyde.

(2) Mania often induces pressured speech so that patients incessantly talk, either face-to-face or over the phone (often making numerous phone calls). The patient's voice

may be loud and difficult to understand due to its rapidity. I am one of the few who are sometimes able to control this symptom when in mania, although I have gone on calling rampages several times due to manic episodes. The content of speech commonly reflects an authoritative view that supercedes anyone else on all subjects. Furthermore the patient has a strong desire to verbalize this "knowledge." This therefore contributes to, and reinforces, the pressure of the speech. I have often been told that in the manic state "you don't sound like yourself."

(3) A person who is manic will often be distracted by, or place significance in, things that others would typically not notice: for instance a fly landing on a leaf or the movement of a cloud. Because of a heightened religious state (referred to as hyperreligiosity, a feature often observed in bipolar disorder), I would note these as symbols of order in the universe and definite signs from God to me. For example, I might take particular notice of a passing truck while in the midst of a conversation. I would then read the words displayed on its exterior and derive a meaning that was totally ludicrous. Thus, if the passing vehicle had the words "Wisconsin Dairy

Farm" on it, I would interpret this as a sign that the individual I was interacting with was going to move to a farm in Wisconsin to raise cows.

(4) When manic, a person may become extremely goal-oriented. At school he might be seen studying several hours more per day in pursuit of a perfect grade point average. If employed, an exceptional devotion to work on a specific project may develop. A patient's driven behavior may also be exhibited socially by increasing attendance at parties, political gatherings, church or other public venues in an attempt to elevate his status in the community. Another symptom will be a sudden, highly focused or overbearing drive to develop an intimate relationship with another person(s). This may be due to an increased sexual drive. Extensive planning may occur in more than one of these goal-directed endeavors at the same time. In all of these cases the goal(s) will usually be significantly, if not totally, misguided. Unfortunately, I have exhibited all of these phenomena. As is typical for most people who suffer from a manic episode, I felt a deep pain afterward because of my actions and this contributed to the major depression that invariably followed.

This fourth symptom can be considered ful-filled as well if the patient is restless, agitated or can't stand still for more than a moment (medically termed hyperactivity or more pre-cisely psychomotor agitation). I had bound-less energy, often uncontrolled, when manic. I would walk for miles, sometimes for no par-ticular reason, to no destination, at any hour of the day or night. I would also play tennis interminably, compared to my healthy state, without tiring.

(5) Another symptom is excessive behav-ior, usually in the pursuit of pleasure, that is likely to have painful consequences. Examples include buying sprees beyond financial ability, promiscuity, foolish business ventures and risky high-speed driving. With my unbridled energy and euphoria I some-times shopped endlessly and purchased items that were completely unnecessary in my non-manic world. Of course, considering myself God, I knew that I owned everything anyway. Fortunately, despite my elevated sex drive, I did not participate in any indiscriminate sexu-al activity. My chaste values are deeply held such that they probably kept me from acting on those manic desires. Nonetheless, when Mr. Hyde is present even deeply held values

can be inverted. I was also fortunate in that I did not engage in any foolish business ventures that are common to others with the illness. In medical school it was related to me how one man invested in thousands of toilet seats. However, I believed I could win a million dollars in professional tennis and that my degrees were worthless. Indeed, I discarded all of my diplomas on one occasion.

In my first hospitalization I met a mother and daughter who both had the disease and were manic at the same time. They described a dangerous game of "chicken," during which they would occupy both lanes of a two-lane highway. I briefly questioned the reality of much of life, let alone the rules of the road, and was considering driving without regard to any laws, but luckily did not do so. Traveling to distant cities without contacting anyone is a common manifestation of mania. I left town on many occasions; sometimes with a destination in mind and at other instances to nowhere in particular, as an impulsive byproduct of my increased energy state. Many times it entered my mind to travel to Hawaii, which I actually fulfilled as Ira discussed in Chapter 1.

There is also an appearance change (facial expression, hairstyle, dress, etc.) that frequently reflects or accompanies the personality transformation. I looked markedly different, with extreme weight loss to 98 pounds, and growth of long hair for the first and only time in my life during one manic episode. This again might suggest the transformation of Dr. Jekyll to Mr. Hyde.

At this point I want to reemphasize that these behavior patterns were extremely different from my normal personality. In my euthymic, or normal state, I am a very deliberate, comparison shopper, one of the most cautious drivers on the road and particular about my appearance.

(6) Another symptom, termed the flight of ideas, is the rapid passing from one subject to another, for example, talking about cars, then suddenly a recipe, then computers, politics, etc. Though the topics may be diverse there is usually a connection between the thoughts to the patient. I had this thought pattern several times but rarely did I exhibit this in my speech such that a psychiatrist would be able to observe it.

(7) A decreased need for sleep often develops. When ill, the manic person may feel rested even though he has had only two hours of sleep for the night. Sometimes he

does not sleep at all. On many occasions I must have appeared like a caged animal in the hospital when I would stay awake throughout the entire night pacing back and forth. I have observed this behavior in many patients while I was a medical student and resident.

Because of the severity of the mood disturbance, it is thought that daily functioning must be dramatically disrupted or that psychotic (delusions or hallucinations) features must be present to complete the diagnosis of bipolar illness. This may be manifested at work, school or any other social interaction with others (store clerks, ministers, friends, etc.).

A further condition for the diagnosis of mania in the *DSM-IV* is that the symptoms must not be due to drug abuse or an otherwise defined medical disease. Since many people with manic depression self-medicate, the underlying illness may not be immediately evident. They are considered to have a "dual diagnosis" in that they have the diagnoses of substance abuse and manic depression. Alcohol, heroin, cocaine and amphetamines are some of the drugs that may be abused for the purpose of lessening the intensity of a depression or to reproduce the euphoria of mania. I never used any illicit drugs and would drink alcohol only minimally at social occasions and after my diagnosis I completely abstained.

There are a number of other illnesses that can give a clinical picture that could lead to a false diagnosis of manic depression such as head trauma, and kidney or liver disease. For this reason it is important that a complete medical exam be performed as part of the diagnostic process.

The criteria for making the diagnosis for manic depression as set forth in the *DSM-IV* result in a numerical quantity that indicates the presence of the disease. However, in practice, the diagnosis is usually arrived at through the general experience of the physician. In fact, I have never witnessed a psychiatrist explicitly using the *DSM-IV* criteria in the diagnosis of manic depression. This is not surprising, as it is nearly impossible to identify all of the symptoms the patient is suffering from because it is so difficult to know what the patient is thinking at the time of diagnosis. In addition, often only the direct actions that led to the patient being brought to the psychiatrist are known by him (e.g., the police may have caught the individual disturbing the peace, driving recklessly or acting "strange"), not the progression of symptoms described in the *DSM-IV.* These facts draw one to the conclusion that the effort to derive a quantifiable criterion for diagnosis was misdirected because behavior is inherently subjective.

Ira: Stan has described the standard method of diagnosis based on quantifiable measures. If a manic episode does occur, it is extremely difficult for physicians to obtain the medical and family history from the patient. An important point that we will return to in Chapter 4 is that the physician must at least attempt to contact the family to get this information. In fact, if there is one message about diagnosis to emphasize it is that the physician should be humble about his ability to discern the extent of this complex illness with the limited information typically available to him.

Usually the family feels the effects of mania well before any medical help is requested. Even if the patient lives in another city the phone calls Stan described will announce the arrival of Mr. Hyde. The person experiencing manic depressive symptoms is rarely self-aware; thus, it falls on loved ones to recognize the illness before a major episode occurs. As Stan has discussed above, even for professionals diagnosis is problematic, but in my opinion lay people can determine if there is a medical problem even if they cannot pinpoint it. The two key issues to consider are (1) family history and (2) changes in personality.

(1) There is a strong correlation between a family history of mental illness and the appearance of manic depression. However, because of the stigma associated with mental illness, most people do not discuss it, even within their families. If a grandparent was hospitalized, an uncle has committed suicide, a parent was treated by a psychiatrist, if there has been any history of mental illness in a family, I would suggest a heightened awareness among family members for mood disorders. This is especially true for parents of their children. I would discuss the possibility of the onset of mental problems with children at the earliest opportunity.

(2) The key trait to examine in individuals is changes in personality. Virtually all personality traits, certainly moods, can be considered normal or attributed to environmental factors. Any of the behavior patterns described in the *DSM-IV* could be considered normal in isolation. But

significant changes in personality in an individual with a family history of mental illness should be taken very seriously, and include the commencement of professional medical involvement in managing the situation.

Our experience is instructive. Stan and I have always had a good relationship. We did fight as boys when we shared a bedroom, but had hardly had a negative word for each other in years. In our mid-20's this began to change. I went to visit Stan while he was in medical school in Charleston, SC. We had many entertaining activities planned for the week in that charming city. However, he was very irritable and quarrelsome, to the point that I cut short my trip and returned home. I attributed his behavior to the pressures of medical school. In hindsight I realize that this was the first sign of Stan's illness that I had observed. I should have considered my mother's treatment and hospitalization for what had been called a nervous breakdown. In fact, she has suffered from clinical depression and panic disorder for most of her life. But at the time I had no awareness whatsoever of mental illness.

In a sense I am advocating that family members act as *thought police* for each other. I realize this is a negative term for this difficult task, a task with many potential problems because people resent having their thoughts second-guessed. But it is an accurate term. Certainly care and judgement should be exercised before anyone commits someone to the hospital or even initiates psychiatric care. But it is usually only within the family that the change in personality that signals the onset of manic depression can be discerned. Eventually I became highly sensitive to Stan's mania. I could tell when he was manic at first sight by the expression on his face-the face of Mr. Hyde. In speaking with him, even over the phone, I knew almost immediately when Stan was slipping into mania through his topics of discussion and the tone of his voice. Stan described how speech patterns changed and that he could control his at times. I believe now that I could always determine if mania were present even if Stan were trying to mask it.

3. What were the circumstances of your diagnosis?

Stan: I was diagnosed in the fall of 1986 at age 26. A manic episode led to my receiving medical attention and the diagnosis of the disease. My first manic event began in the course of approximately 24 hours. This is in contrast to major depression that is in general far more gradual in onset, possibly beginning with anxiety and melancholia days, weeks or even months earlier. However, prior to this first manic episode I did have indicators of mood instability.

I believe that the symptoms of my illness began in early 1982 when I was 22 years old. Initially I had depressive symptoms that were manifested primarily as periods of increased sleep, but I also had slower thoughts and mild sadness. These would never last more than one or two days. It seemed as though everything would go wrong some days. Sometimes these periods were associated with external events (such as after losing a match in a tennis tournament, catching a cold, underachieving on an exam, being rejected for a date, etc.), but many if not most occurred with no apparent external stimuli. I then developed periods, of slightly shorter duration, when I was somewhat more expansive, jocular, energetic, fast thinking, requiring an hour or two less sleep per night. These would usually occur before tests, oral presentations, new romantic interests, etc. While the depressed days were fraught with disappointment, on these days most, if not all, events were favorable. Even if events did not go well, my heightened emotional state would not allow them to bother me.

The frequency in mood alternation increased with the beginning of medical school. In this environment, learning and testing were very different than in my engineering curriculum of the previous four years. The schedule induced intense studying with clear, quick thinking prior to and during frequent tests, followed by a short interval of relaxation including parties with mild alcohol consumption. Despite this environment, I always did my best to maintain a constant mood, sleep pattern and study methods. Overall I was fairly successful (especially as I became more used to the routine). This does not mean that this environment was not difficult. Sometimes I considered the stress of the tests helpful because it would stimulate me and propel me out of a depressive state.

Besides the depressive symptoms, there was something else on my mind that perplexed and worried me. On a handful of occasions occurring between the completion of the second year of medical school and my first manic episode, I became volatile and/or made statements that were completely uncharacteristic of my normal personality. For example, once at a late hour I awoke and immediately called my eldest brother. I proceeded to criticize him about many aspects of his life in an angry and hostile tone, though I was unaware of my mood. These brief events were unprecedented and I now realize they were a prelude to the mania that was to follow.

I first learned about manic depression through a college psychology course. In medical school it was briefly discussed, but only as an undistinguished morsel in the feast of information I was digesting at that time. I didn't meet the criteria for bipolar disorder or major depression, though I still had some concern, mainly about my depressions. This was in part due to my awareness that my mother suffered from chronic depression for many years such that I had a genetic predisposition to major depression. Thus, my medical training only provided me limited insight to foresee the onset of my illness.

The manic episode began with increased thoughts of religion and a general increase in energy. I began to attend a Baptist church that had many young members, some of them being students at the Medical University. Previously I never had actively practiced any religion, only occasionally attending church with friends, in part to be sociable as well as to expand my knowledge and experience of others. At this time, however, I began attending by myself. During the sermons my mind wandered to the stained glass and thoughts that I was "special." I listened to the songs in honor of Christ and thought that they were directed toward me. I even went to the Sunday school, something I had never even considered before. This was totally spontaneous and was the beginning of my loss of self-determination and control.

Eventually my mood became volatile, with a rapid progression of thoughts. My emotions alternated from the deepest sadness, connected to thoughts of the death of loved ones (not in any specific detail, but as if I could predict the end of their lives), to a joviality in which I discovered something outlandishly humorous in events that I had never put any significance in before (some of them from the distant past). To recognize the humor, I thought, required a keen insight and interpretive abilities others did not possess. These rapid mood swings affected my behavior. I drove aimlessly to several churches. I stopped going to school, where at this time I was doing physiology research for my Ph.D.

I developed a strange sense of fear. It seemed as though everyone were behaving unusually because, I thought, the end of time was near. For a few moments I began driving recklessly at high speeds and ignoring stop signs as though it would not place my life at risk (normally I am a very careful driver). I was sleeping fewer hours especially when compared to the minor depressions I had been experiencing. I became obsessed with photography. I thought I could discern the true essence of an individual I did not know merely from his or her image on the film. In general I felt as though I understood the world to a degree that no one else had ever done before. In effect, I believed that I understood the reason for "everything."

My illness became apparent to my family when I called them in the middle of the night for no reason. Ira traveled from Durham, NC to see what was happening and I told him to leave without letting him in my apartment. At that time I spoke in an angry tone, but actually had no particular emotion. Later I went to a neighbor's door and, with no motive, unaware of my mood (like sleep-walking but awake), took a wreath off her door and threw it to the ground. I also set my dog loose and placed all of his food, heart worm pills and grooming supplies in the trash. The neighbor whose wreath I tossed called the police, who then came to my residence. I began crying, which was unusual for me, but without feeling any sadness. While in the presence of the police I called my best friend from college. They did not speak to my friend but apparently the conversation made them believe that my behavior was now under control and I was not dangerous to anyone, even though in hindsight I recall that part of the dialogue was very strange. For example, I told him about the significance of colors, yellow representing peace, red being blood, etc.

After two more days absence from school my academic advisor and mentor called me at home. It was a very short conversation, as I felt numb. I was no longer grandiose, but now very tired. He asked me to come to school and without argument I agreed. Upon arrival he gave me the name and phone number of a psychiatrist and suggested I call him. I had great respect for my advisor as well as a strong friendship with him, and thus followed his advice. This was the first time in my life I had sought professional help for a psychiatric or behavioral disorder.

The psychiatrist was very casual in appearance such that he did not look like other academicians to me. He was gracious and stated that all of his notes would stay in his office and remain confidential. I told him a synopsis of what had occurred. He proceeded to give me a mini-mental-status exam that consisted of naming the town in which I lived, reciting the names of recent presidents, basic mathematics, interpreting proverbs, etc. I answered all of the questions normally. His assessment was that something unusual (idiosyncratic) had happened or that I had manic depression. He went on to say that manic depression is a good diagnosis to have, because if it were responsible for my behavior, lithium could control my symptoms. He also had me complete a psychological test called the Minnesota Multiphasic Personality Inventory. This consists of written responses to 550 statements that are designed to indicate abnormalities in personality. The results of this test did not reveal clear evidence of an elevated mood state called hypomania that often accompanies the illness. He reassured me that nobody would have taken much notice of my recent behavior, and that I should not concern myself with the consequences of my actions beyond apologizing to my neighbor and any others I may have encountered.

I was stable for the next three weeks, then my energy again increased while my sleep declined. I went into school at night, where a brief conversation with my fellow graduate students ensued. They told me later that they noticed my behavior was unusual. I returned to my apartment for the evening. I was hyperreligious to such a degree that in the middle of the night I impulsively called the airlines, though there was no answer, to get a flight to Israel, which I believed was my true homeland. I did not attempt to schedule this trip again. In the morning I returned to school. I walked throughout the hospital in a euphoric state. Eventually I ended up in the office of another one of my academic advisors. He realized that I was ill, so he escorted me to the psychiatrist's office. I was given a prescription for lithium. When I left the psychiatrist's office I immediately tore up the prescription. Early the following morning

I impulsively drove my car to the airport. I left it in the drop-off lane and walked to the ticket counter. I asked for a flight to Hawaii but the agent did not oblige. I then walked to one of the gates and sat down in the empty airport. A security officer arrived, handcuffed me, and took me to a room where I spoke filthy language to her. It is extremely unusual for me to use profane language; furthermore, I had no internal emotion at that time. I was speaking but was unconscious of my thoughts. I was taken to the hospital and was seen by another psychiatrist who made the diagnosis of bipolar disorder. After waiting in the emergency room for several hours I was brought to the psychiatric ward. It was locked so that patients could not leave without permission. When the psychiatry resident arrived he placed me in a private, locked cell because my mood had become aggravated. He gave me a brief physical exam and then called security to hold me down in order to draw blood (this was done to test for other medical diseases that might have been affecting my behavior) and began treatment by injecting an antipsychotic drug.

Ira: During the events described by Stan, my mother, our brother Mike, and myself were overwhelmed by indecision. We knew something was wrong with him from his late-night phone calls. His advisor also called, informing me of Stan's erratic behavior. So it was obvious something was very wrong with Stan, but we had no knowledge of mental illness. For virtually any other illness I could have initiated treatment in some way, but for mental illness we had no idea what to do. Handling Mr. Hyde is a difficult task. As noted earlier in the Preface, it is precisely to provide a resource for families in the same predicament that we wrote this book.

At this time I was attending Duke University in Durham, North Carolina. I went to the school psychologist for advice. After a short description of the situation he suggested that Stan was schizophrenic and that there was nothing I could do. This discussion was the first of many I would have over the years with psychologists and psychiatrists. Needless to say my experience has formed in me a strong opinion about their abilities, which I shall discuss in Chapter 4.

I was in despair, for it seemed I had lost my brother to something I did not understand. But I felt I must try to see for myself at least how Stan appeared physically, and to see if our family dog living with him was all right. I left in the early evening on a Friday, driving about six hours down to Charleston, and arrived sometime after midnight. For some reason my sensibilities kept me from ringing Stan's bell in the middle of the night, so I waited in the car, sleeping when possible, until morning. At about eight I rang Stan's door. He opened the door but he would not talk to me. At the first instance I could perceive something was different, even if I did not understand that it was the face of Mr. Hyde. But he appeared physically sound and I could see that our dog was alive and well. At that point I did not see anything more I could do in Charleston. So after that 15-second encounter I got back in my car and drove back to Durham.

For the next couple of days I was contemplating and looking into the procedure for getting Stan committed to a hospital. At that time I could not get any useful information. However, the tension was relieved when that first manic episode broke and Stan went to see the psychiatrist. Stan called me to explain that it was probably the niacin he was taking (to lower his cholesterol) that caused his erratic behavior. It was certainly good to hear Stan's voice again as opposed to Hyde's. Unfortunately, this pleasant experience would have to be repeated many more times in the future.

As Stan has described, three weeks later he relapsed into mania. I received a message from his advisor that there was an emergency and that Stan was missing. Once again I drove down to Charleston, not knowing what I would find there. Thankfully he was in the hospital when I arrived. For the first time I heard the term "manic depression" from the psychiatrist treating Stan. Searching my memory, the only other occasion on which I could recall hearing the term was from an episode of the sitcom *Maude*, hardly a source for the kind of information I needed. This was the beginning of my education.

In a cell-like room in the psychiatric ward of the hospital Stan appeared and acted possessed. This was especially the case when the attendants forcibly injected him with medication in an attempt to end his psychosis. Watching that scene was the one point in all of our trials and tribulations where I felt fear, fear about what would happen to Stan and how my family would be able to cope with it. I have come to realize that it was my inexperience and ignorance of the disease that caused my trepidation. It is a lack of knowledge that can make a difficult situation a hopeless one.

4. What causes manic depression?

Stan: As with many diseases, the cause of manic depression must be considered within the spectrum of nature vs. nurture. In other words, the interaction between genetic factors and something specific in the environment is responsible for causing it. Family studies reveal that those who have a parent or sibling (first-degree relatives) with the disease have a ten-fold greater risk of developing the illness themselves than if the illness were not present within the family, even if raised in different environments (adopted by different parents at birth). If an identical twin has the disease, there is a 75% likelihood that the other twin, with the exact same genetic composition, will have bipolar disorder. Conversely, because 25% of the time one twin will not develop manic depression, some other factor(s) in the environment must be necessary for the illness to be manifested besides genetic predisposition.

In an attempt to understand the genetic basis for the disease, researchers over the past several years have investigated families in which the illness is clustered; however, there has been no identification of the specific genes and chromosomes that determine if one is predisposed to manic depression. Finding the inheritance pattern for manic depression is difficult because it is not a simple correlation like that for eye color in fruit flies, which you might have studied in your high school biology class. The color of the eye is determined by whether or not a dominant gene is present in a specific pair of chromosomes. In humans, diseases such as sickle cell anemia (a blood disorder) and Huntington's disease (a neurologic illness) are genetically inherited due to chromosomal abnormalities of a single gene, thus it is possible in these cases for genetic screening to detect the source of the disease.

The genetics of manic depression are far more complex. Finding the genes is inherently difficult because the diagnosis of manic depression itself is clinical and not objective (again, no blood or imaging test for it exists). No single gene causes the illness; in bipolar disorder, a number of genes, possibly on different chromosomes, may interact to determine if one has the predisposition to develop the symptoms. This is similar to patterns of inheritance called polygenic inheritance, which also applies to the passing of intelligence and height. To add more complexity to the matter, bipolar disorder may actually be a conglomerate of several illnesses, with different genes responsible for each one.

The degree to which the environment causes manic depression is just as difficult to determine. For example, events that make a person happy or elevate one's mood may lead the predisposed individual to euphoria and subsequent mania. Other likely factors which affect the onset of mania include sleep deprivation (the quantity and quality of sleep are very important in this disease), the season (thought to be more common in the spring), work-related pressure and various emotional stressors such as relationship problems. On the opposite pole, events that lower your mood can trip one who is susceptible into a major depressive episode. It is also possible that the resolution of a depression may directly precipitate a manic episode.

Other environmental factors that cause the expression of the illness are not so clear. Nevertheless, these could be more important, particularly in those with no apparent genetic predisposition. Examples might include fear of abandonment at a critical age as a result of parental neglect, high blood pressure while in the womb, deficiency of a dietary substance as an infant, a specific viral infection, etc. Needless to say, comprehending all the factors that induce manic depression is a daunting task.

5. What are your risk factors for manic depression?

Stan: To reiterate, the causes of bipolar disorder are uncertain but are certainly related to complex combinations of genetic factors and environmental influences. The environmental sources may be readily identifiable or quite obscure. Each person has to individually analyze and try to attenuate or mitigate the effects of likely outside factors that precipitate his symptoms. I have listed what I consider the likely factors that have caused my illness below.

We know of no family member who had manic depression. However, as noted earlier, my mother did have a history of psychiatric problems. She clearly was afflicted with recurrent major depressive disorder. This increased my risk of developing bipolar disorder, because a family history of other mental illnesses, especially the unipolar mood disorder major depression, elevates the risk of having manic depression. She has also suffered from another psychiatric illness: severe anxiety due to panic disorder.

Environmental factors that probably contributed to my symptoms were sleep deprivation, emotional work pressures-primarily at institutions that were not supportive-not being settled in a permanent home and job, and not being married, as I desired.

Ira: Because the effects of the organic illness and environmental experiences cannot be separated, there is no way to know for sure what initiates a particular manic episode. As an engineer and scientist I understand that the difficulty in pinpointing a cause exists because no controlled experiments are possible. For example, we have thought that the high pressure and sleep deprivation associated with Stan's medical training might have initiated some of his manic episodes. But we cannot turn back time and put an identical Stan into a different situation to test that hypothesis. There is no way to know for sure. A related concept is what I call the nonlinearity of manic depression. We naturally find ourselves extrapolating Stan's history, or the his-

tory of other patients, to some future consequence. Imagine extending a line forward to
predict a future data point. But manic depression is not a line. Every case is different and
every point in time is different for each person.
The lack of controlled experiments and the
inherent non-linearity of manic depression make
the study and treatment of it extremely difficult.
Virtually this entire book is colored by these
facts.

6. What do you think about and what do you do
during a manic episode?

Stan: When manic I was usually euphoric, though I have also been angry. My self-
control is lost, as I am not aware of the implications of my actions. My thoughts have run
the gamut from ecstasy to primal fear. For
example, as "God" I thought I was ushering
a perfect world into being. On another occasion, when being taken to the hospital, I
thought I was being escorted to my wedding.
What a surprise upon crossing the threshold!
I have also felt fear due to the belief that my
own death and those of loved ones was
imminent. Although thoughts about death
are usually more common with depression,

they can be observed in mania as well. I did not contemplate suicide during any of my manic periods but I can conceive of it being possible given what my mind was enduring. It was like I was spinning in a circle, unable to focus on a destination, and going nowhere. I would literally become nauseated such that only falling asleep relieved the discomfort.

7. What do you think about and what do you do during hypomania?

Stan: Hypomania is the main defining characteristic of Bipolar II disorder. Thus far I have been describing when a manic period exists in Bipolar I disorder. Hypomania is a less severe form of mania. In the *DSM-IV* a hypomanic episode is described as a persistent, elevated, expansive or irritable change in mood, as compared to the nondepressed mood, lasting at least four consecutive days. The comparison to the nondepressed mood may be difficult because depressions can last months or years. Thus, the normal, nondepressed mood may not be recognizable to the patient or his loved ones. At least three (four if in the irritable mood state) of the symptoms described for a manic episode must be present to a significant degree to designate a hypomanic state. Recall that these are (1) increased self-esteem or non-delusional grandiosity, (2) decreased sleep, (3) pressured, incessant speech, (4) easy distractibility, (5) rapid thoughts, (6) increased goal-directed activities or agitation and (7) involvement in pleasurable activities likely to have painful consequences.

The disturbance in mood and change in functioning must be observable by others. This is a loaded criterion because of course the "others" need to have known the person in the past. Furthermore, they must be familiar with that individual's personality and have interacted with him frequently enough to realize the current alteration. Even then, it can still be difficult to discern this change. Mood is not always prominently displayed even if one is disturbed. It may be necessary to speak with and observe the hypomanic person for several hours before the symptoms become apparent.

In contrast to a manic episode, the symptoms of hypomanic episodes are not severe enough to cause a marked impairment in social or occupational function.

Hospitalization is not usually required, but the individual can still harm himself because of his behavior-e.g., financial loss, damage to reputation, etc. There are no psychotic aspects to a hypomanic episode where psychosis usually consists of losing touch with reality with hallucinations, e.g., hearing voices or seeing things that are not physically present and/or having delusions. Similar to a manic event, the symptoms are not due to the direct effects of drugs, toxins or a general medical condition.

I have experienced many periods of elevated, expansive (rarely have I been irritable) mood states that met or partially met the criteria for a hypomanic episode. These occurred more frequently than the manic episodes and predated the first mania by years. I believe that the more unstable my mood with respect to depressive, and especially hypomanic states, the greater the probability for a future manic event. Although I may have seemed more vivacious during them, my hypomanic moods were not pleasant or desirable to me.

Many individuals state that they wish for these episodes. I prefer to have more control and stability. I felt wired or too hyped up to the point of being uncomfortable. Friends on occasion observed this and commented that I was acting unusual because of my increased talking and elevated mood. My behavior was similar to the lack of inhibition associated with alcohol consumption. For example, I would laugh, tell jokes, and be more humorous than usual. I did not suffer to any major degree from these hypomanic states besides restless sleep unless it led to full mania. As with manic episodes, following the period of decreased sleep I often would have a period of increased sleep.

Some people claim that during hypomania they have increased creativity, rapidity and clarity of thought, and, thus, an increase in productivity. For short periods (less than 48 hours) I did experience this, seeming to accomplish a great deal. For example, I might wake as much as two hours early, work 12-14 hours with what appeared to be higher concentration, shop for groceries, wash my car, clean my apartment (cleaning was nearly always a component of my elevated mood states), do the laundry, play two hours of competitive singles tennis, and then go out on a date (with increased sexual drive). However, overall the thoughts were too rapid and my patience was reduced, negating any perceived gain. Eventually there would be a net loss in productivity because my mood would eventually cycle downward.

8. How was mania manifested in your thoughts?

Stan: I have described some of my actions while manic. Here I will describe what I was thinking while manic. A very different person inhabits my body during a manic episode, i.e., Mr. Hyde. I cannot describe all of these thoughts, though I shall describe those that were pervasive and particular for me, and those that are common to some others in the manic state. Most of these thoughts were delusions, literally false beliefs. I hope that by presenting some of the finer details of my experience with the illness, other patients can better relate to the manifestations of the disease and families can understand the madness to a greater extent.

Hyperreligiosity: I was never one to participate in organized religion or even think much about God. I experienced a sudden change when I became manic. As noted earlier, I attended church services alone for the first time, probably as part of my expansive state. As I sat in the pew I felt that I was Jesus Christ, even though I knew little about the Bible or Jesus. Within days I was stating that I was God. The belief that I was God at times made me euphoric. However, I also became deeply saddened and/or over-whelmed with fear and persecutory delusions on other occasions, as I became preoccupied with the crucifixion. I felt that it was I who had experienced the mocking, beating and hanging that Christ endured.

During my last major manic episode I developed a rationale about why I was God, namely that nobody but God could have an M.D., a Ph.D., be the greatest athlete in the world, and look as stunning as myself. I told nearly everyone I met that I was God. I became angry if I felt that an individual denied or did not comprehend my state-ments. Several other delusions were also dan-gerous. For instance, I thought that it was necessary and important to look directly into the sun. Only I understood that this gave people unlimited energy by absorption of photons. In addition, I alone was able to eat a diet of just flour and water, based on the Biblical account of the exodus from Egypt.

As another example, I drove with the belief that cars didn't need gasoline or oil. In accordance with my beliefs I was authoritative and would tell people that they should follow everything I did. I would not validate or accept anyone else's views on anything-I always had to have the last word. I envisioned everyone as children with myself as an all-knowing father.

As part of my hyperreligiosity I watched religious television stations in the belief that this was a method for me to hear people's prayers. I read through the entire Bible three or four times in order to know it thoroughly. Of course delusions need not be consistent, so it did not bother me that if I were God I wouldn't need to read the Bible to know it.

I believed that I preprogrammed the universe millions of years ago so that all events, including miracles, would occur precisely when necessary. As part of this plan, I made myself human with no extraordinary powers other than my incomparable knowledge. Thus, I humbled myself extraordinarily by becoming human, my spirit being the God of all the ages-the one who spoke to Abraham and Moses. Everything I did was perfect and I wanted everyone to realize this and to praise and worship me. I believed that I could not be harmed by any weapon, therefore, when not in the paranoid phase of my disease, I felt invulnerable and immortal.

I developed an urge to write during some of my manic episodes. In the last one, when I thought I was God, I felt it was incumbent on me as a benevolent deity to document the way to a perfect universe in a pamphlet.

Grandiose thoughts: As I have just elaborated in regard to my hyperreligiosity, I had the ultimate grandiose thought in believing that I was God. I attended church services with the belief that they were conducted to honor me. I also had other grandiose thoughts that were delusional. It was my belief that I was the greatest tennis player in the world and could defeat any pro. I then devised a scheme to demonstrate my ability. I faxed an application to the United States Tennis Association to play in tournaments to display my miraculous talent. I actually played in some satellite tournaments. I was trounced in my matches but never wavered in my delusion that I was the best-my excuse for losing being that it wasn't the appropriate time to reveal my ability. My mission was to teach everyone in the world how to play because tennis was such a beneficial sport and I was the perfect one to emulate playing it.

To a lesser degree, I had grandiose thoughts that I could sing better than anyone else did. Music was a frequent component of my hypomanic and manic episodes. I would often play it loud and found hidden meanings in the lyrics. Another grandiose thought was that both my cooking skills and acting abilities were second to none. Furthermore, I believed my knowledge of science and mathematics was miraculous. I would explain any action in terms of scientific theories: the laws of thermodynamics, Einstein's theory of relativity, etc.

Buying sprees and throwing out possessions: Buying sprees almost always accompanied my manic episodes, I personified the slogan "shop till you drop." I loved going to malls. Some of my purchases were expensive, but cost was no concern because of my euphoria. On two occasions I bought an engagement ring for women who were no more than casual friends. I once purchased a house, making an offer at the listed price with no other negotiation. This price was well above the true market value. Incredibly, I bought a new car when I was unemployed and signed for the car as "God." However, I primarily bought clothes, usually just after discarding most of my existing wardrobe. Throwing things out seemed to be due to an internal drive to clean that went wildly awry. At other times I threw out the clothes because I believed it was time to dispense with everything associated with the past, including photographs, trophies, textbooks and diplomas. I rationalized this behavior based on the New Testament, where Jesus told the rich man to give away his personal possessions.

Paranoia: In many instances I experienced a feeling of paranoia from which specific sources of anxiety would develop. Examples included fear of getting fired from my job, that the police were after me, and, most dreadfully, the perceived persecution that I was to be hanged for being Jesus Christ (my hyperreligiosity). In 1995 I purchased the album *The Lion King* since I thought I was the "King." The instrumental music generated immense fear in me, as though it were specifically composed to make me lose all semblance of reality. I continuously felt the presence of death. In my mind I experienced the horror of dying in every conceivable manner, including getting buried alive, drowning, suffering a life-ending heart attack and being struck on the head with a hammer. I thought waitresses were poisoning my drinks and the police were going to shoot me. I believed my residence was the site of many murders and my neighbors were responsible for many assassinations. I was living in a realm I never want to reenter-it was more emotionally terrifying than any movie or book that I have ever heard of.

Late-night phone calls: Normally I rarely awakened during the night, but during manic episodes I had a propensity for phone calls. My calling rampages were spontaneous and done with an angry tone, though sometimes my inner feelings can best be described as numb or without an appreciation for my behavior. In other cases I felt genuine anger because I thought I was being treated unfairly, especially in being taken to a hospital and locked in a ward. The calling periods were usually nocturnal and consisted of speech that was totally uncharacteristic of my normal speech. It was loud, rapid, lewd and profane. It was and remains almost impossible for me to believe it was I saying those things.

I would make as many as 15 of these calls in immediate succession before taking a break, then calling again.

9. What were your depressions like?

Stan: Depression is the mood at the opposite end of the spectrum from mania. Major depressive disorder is the unipolar mood disorder. There is thought to be some relationship between bipolar disorder and major depressive disorder in that if one has a relative with depression, one has an increased risk of developing manic depression. Moreover, many of those who are originally diagnosed with major depressive disorder will later develop manic depression. A major depressive episode can be just as debilitating as a manic episode but in a different manner.

In order to put my symptoms into context, it is instructive to present the definition and criteria employed to diagnose a major depressive episode according to the *DSM-IV*. Since most people have experienced the blues or mild depression, this diagnosis is easier to relate to than the symptoms of a manic episode.

Depression is a change in function over at least a two-week period with a depressed mood or loss of interest or pleasure in usual pursuits. This consists of five or more of nine possible symptoms in this clinical guideline.

(1) A depressed mood most of the day for most days.
(2) Significant losses of pleasure in most, if not all activities.
(3) Decrease in appetite with associated weight loss or an increased appetite with weight gain, totaling a 5% change in body weight over the course of a month.
(4) Increased sleep (hypersomnia) or decreased sleep (insomnia) almost every day.
(5) Restlessness or inability to sit still (psychomotor agitation) or the opposite (psychomotor retardation) nearly every day.
(6) Fatigue or loss of energy almost every day.
(7) Feelings of worthlessness or extreme guilt almost every day.
(8) Decreased ability to concentrate or think nearly every day.

(9) Recurrent thoughts of death and suicide. This includes contemplation of what the loss of the individual's life would mean. There may or may not be a concrete plan for actually committing suicide.

In addition to the symptoms listed above, there must be a significant disruption in the individual's life with respect to social, occupational or other important functions. The symptoms displayed must not be due to drugs of any kind or any other medical condition. Furthermore, clinical depression should not be diagnosed if the symptoms occur in relation to the loss of a loved one. Technically, this would be called bereavement.

I have experienced depression innumerable times from mild melancholia to an almost comatose, vegetative state. As I mentioned previously, at least since 1982 I began experiencing depressions. But none of these early episodes met the *DSM-IV* criteria for a major depressive episode. Nevertheless, they had an impact on my life. My symptoms of depression have generally been more prominent in the mornings, the increased sleep making it difficult to wake up. These depressions would generally last only 24-48 hours but increased in length as the years went by. At times they would be frequent, for one depressive state might occur within one week of a previous episode. There have been external circumstances that have been associated with my depressions. However, I also believe I have suffered from depressions due to no external circumstances. The contradictory and confusing nature of cause and effect are hallmarks of mental illness.

The predominant symptom of my depressions was an increased need for sleep. Sometimes there were sad feelings and a decreased ability to concentrate associated with this fatigue. When the sadness fell in with my minor depressions, I felt an emptiness and loneliness. I would ruminate on and amplify my problems, even old and insignificant ones. Most people were unaware of my discomfort. I never mentioned my problems because I didn't think discussing them would help me. It did amaze me that, as far as I knew, nobody was aware of how tired and low I really was, but I was pleased that it was not apparent.

In contrast to the minor depressive episodes, after my manic episodes in 1991,

1994 and 1995 I suffered severe depressions to the extent that I was in a near vegetative state. The weight of the depressions was so great that my mind actually turned off, putting me into a deep sleep. This never lasted very long, however. As I would awake, emotional and physical pain would ensue. The physical pain was essentially due to my mind-state and never worse than in 1991 when my entire body felt as though I had extreme sunburn. Furthermore, I was constantly nauseated. Despite the nausea, I developed a craving for fast food that I don't have at other times. During my depressions I usually have an elevated appetite. This hunger along with the decreased activity in the depressed state resulted in weight gain. In some ways this would compensate for the weight loss that occurred during the increased energy period associated with the preceding mania. However, my weight gain has overcompensated and increased significantly over my normal body weight, returning to normal only with the end of the depression. The emotional pain arose from both an underlying, nondescript discomfort as well as a focus on what I had lost (including my job and the realization that the perfect world I had envisioned was not real). I experienced uncontrollable crying spells. I had no pleasure in life at this time. It was a burden to perform the most basic daily tasks, such as bathing, shaving, brushing my teeth or getting dressed. I did not even have the ability to read a newspaper or watch TV.

I was extremely grateful coming out of depressions (even the small ones) because I felt that I would never escape their grip while experiencing them. Each time I recovered from a depression I felt a great appreciation for health (even before the diagnosis I considered these sleepy periods a non-defined form of illness). I would attempt to make this time as productive as possible because I was certain another minor depression with increased sleep and melancholy would follow. I think that going through these low emotional states has made me significantly more sensitive and compassionate to others experiencing health problems.

Coming out of the major depressions was far more dramatic. First, there was the seemingly miraculous rapid disappearance of pain and nausea. Other improvements would quickly follow. Now food, even raw vegetables, had immense flavor. I was more aware of my surroundings. To continue the improvement in health required exercise. I usually love and crave exercise, but it became arduous during depressions. The more I exercised the more the depression would abate. It thus seems that for myself to be in optimum mental health without depressive symptoms, I require strenuous exercise at least two or three days a week. The reader should recognize, however, that exercise alone does not necessarily treat or prevent depressions.

10. Have you ever had suicidal thoughts?

Stan: This is a very significant question because some studies reveal that individuals with manic depression have a 15 times greater risk of suicide than the general population. It is generally accepted that if a patient is asked if he has any thoughts of hurting himself an honest answer and dialogue will follow. However, as Ira stressed in the question on making the diagnosis of bipolar disorder, the psychiatrist must also be humble about his ability to prevent patients self-inflicted harm, including suicide. This is true even in the controlled environment of a hospital.

Suicidal thoughts have not been a prominent component of my depressions, even during the severe episodes. In 1992 I did experience a brief impulsive thought of death during the transition from hospitalization to discharge. Following one week in the hospital, I was released during the day to readjust to the outside world and handle my affairs, but was required to return to the hospital for the night. At this time I still had some symptoms of mania (especially the increased energy as well as poor judgment) and some of depression (disappointment over my hospitalization and the reality of the resulting problems). On the first day of the day-pass period I came upon a bridge over the interstate on the way to my apartment and thought for a split second about jumping to my death. I had had no previous contemplation of suicide, but at that moment I had an empty feeling. This demonstrates how difficult it is for anyone, including a psychiatrist, to predict and prevent the occurrence of such an act. This suicidal thought was the closest I have come to purposely killing myself even though on other occasions I felt far more depressed.

In contrast to thought of suicide in the depressive state, when I was manic I almost lost my life because of my irrational behavior, the most notable example being my afore-mentioned disregard for some of the rules of the road. In one manic episode I drove with-out glasses or contact lenses even though I am nearsighted, thinking that this was the way we are supposed to see or that my vision would return to normal.

chapter three:

the pharmacology of manic depression

Chronic mental illnesses, in particular manic depression, are now treated primarily with medications. A common misconception is that simply taking these medications will control or even cure mental disorders. For example, on television shows it is implied that if patients would only take their medications they would be symptom-free. Actually, none of these drugs can be considered a magic bullet, and they must always be supplemented with regular observation and support of the patient by loved ones. Nonetheless, drug therapy is widely prescribed by psychiatrists, and thus it is imperative for patients and families to understand the pharmacology of the medications to some extent. This chapter is designed to provide an introduction to this complicated subject in order to maximize the likelihood for success in treatment when medication is introduced. Initially I describe some of the fundamentals of the brain, what is known about the chemistry of the disease and how medications affect that chemistry. The definition of drug "effectiveness" is then addressed. Next I present short descriptions of common drugs utilized in manic depression and, where applicable, my personal experiences with them. A concluding section then discusses issues related to the implementation of medications in general and how this applies to manic depression.

The Brain

To understand the pharmacology used for the treatment of manic depression, it is important to first understand some facts about the brain. This is because it is within this organ that emotion and thoughts are derived and, therefore, where the medications must act directly, or possibly indirectly, to be effective. The brain is the control center of the human body. The lower portion or brainstem controls basic bodily functions such as respiration and heart rate. The upper area is more complex. It is here that consciousness and emotions are developed, though the specific mechanisms are not understood. The structure of the brain begins with the basic unit of the nervous system, the nerve cell or neuron. There are 100 billion nerve cells in the brain. These cells receive information from other neurons, process the input, and subsequently pass along output messages. Communication between neurons occurs at the region known as the synapse. Any of several messenger molecules such as dopamine, serotonin and norepinephrine may operate within the synapse.

Mechanisms of Disease and Medication

The predominant theories of manic depression are based on the assumption that there is a chemical imbalance in the brain. The term is not specific but it does point to a pathologic condition. The abnormality is thought to reside in the synapse, and is manifested as either an overabundance or deficiency in the concentration (more precisely activity) of chemical messengers. This results in a malfunction in nerve communication. The pharmacological treatment of manic depression is based on the postulate that correcting the chemical imbalance with medications should relieve the patient of symptoms.

The function, or malfunction, of dopamine is now believed to maintain a key role in mental illnesses including manic depression. It is speculated that increased levels of dopamine produce psychotic thoughts such as delusions and hallucinations. Drugs that inhibit dopamine activity, antipsychotics, are thus believed to restore normal thoughts. In addition to the role of dopamine in psychosis, the chemical messengers serotonin and norepinephrine are considered important in the depressive phase of bipolar disorder. Most antidepressants are theorized to act by increasing the low concentration of these messengers in the synapse.

As relatively simple as this concept of a chemical imbalance may appear, it is important to reemphasize that emotions are physiologically complex and the precise locations and mechanisms are still only minimally understood. Unfortunately, I have found through my experience as a patient, that psychiatrists often accept the mechanism models as dogma, as opposed to the actual modest understanding of these complex phenomena. This is not meant to demean the potential benefit of medications and the physicians who prescribe them but rather to put in proper perspective their current utility.

Drug Effectiveness and Side Effects

Several groups of medications are now available for the treatment and control of different manifestations of bipolar disorder. The primary pharmacological agents are the mood stabilizers, antipsychotics and antidepressants. General guidelines exist but pharmacological treatment with respect to the drugs prescribed and the respective dosages must be determined individually for each patient. None of these medicines are effective in all people. Some people may respond to one drug and not another in the same class. It is often deemed necessary to use several drugs because a variety of symptoms persist. This is not only to achieve effectiveness against the illness, but also because secondary medications may be required to counter side effects induced by the primary drugs. The degree of effectiveness, irrespective of whether one or more drugs are used, is also quite variable.

The very definition of effective is open to debate because it is extremely difficult to ascertain. Most fundamentally, effectiveness in reducing manic/depressive symptoms is determined by subjective evaluation as opposed to clearly defined objective parameters such as blood tests. In my own experience there have been numerous instances when professionals have entirely missed my symptoms. True scientific evaluation requires perfectly matched controls with the exception of one variable. This is theoretically impossible in behavioral studies. Researchers are reduced to perform effectiveness studies comparing populations that come substantially short of attaining this ideal. This does not imply that they are without merit, only that these constraints should be understood. In addition, most drugs are examined for effectiveness over a period of no more than several weeks. Thus, data on long-term (one year or more) use are difficult to find in the literature. This is understandable considering the problems, such as prohibitive cost, of such studies. Though on a practical basis, long-term data are crucially important because any relapse can be devastating.

Besides effectiveness, the reported and individual side-effect profiles maintain a major role in determining the medication regimen. For example, a drug that has been found to have toxic effects on the liver in a significant number of patients should not be prescribed to an individual who has a current history of impaired liver function. Similarly, women of childbearing age who may become pregnant must seriously consider taking no medication treatment, termed a "drug holiday," from several of these pharmacological agents utilized in manic depression because of potential fetal toxicity resulting in miscarriages or birth defects.

Bipolar disorder is usually treated with one of the mood stabilizers, drugs that are taken to reduce the propensity for mood swings. If another manic event occurs, the addition of a medication from the other group of mood stabilizers (either lithium or an anticonvulsant as described below) is often added. If further manic breakthroughs occur an antipsychotic will also be administered, because in addition to their primary role in treating psychosis, they are believed to have mood-stabilizing properties. Besides these medications, if depressive symptoms persist, an antidepressant medication may be added with caution (so as to not stimulate the patient into mania) to combat this aspect of the disease.

It should now be apparent that to treat a manic event is not to cure it and that prevention may require manipulation of several drugs at many doses. The dose used is based on standardized blood levels that may be quite arbitrary, the degree of control in any one patient and whether any side effect(s) develops. In order to assess control, and as a primary component of treatment, patients need a close support system to supplement or supercede any drug regimen.

Mood Stabilizers

Lithium was the first medication approved by the Food and Drug Administration (FDA) for the treatment of manic depression as a mood stabilizer. Lithium is a naturally occurring mineral, whereas the anticonvulsant group, including carbamazepime (Tegretol) and valproic acid (Depakote), has more recently been prescribed. Lithium is designated a mood stabilizer by the psychiatric community in that it is thought to minimize fluctuations toward mania and to some extent depression. Despite literally hundreds of studies, the mechanism of lithium in stabilizing the symptoms of manic depression is obscure. Lithium has a number of drawbacks.

It has a narrow therapeutic window, or range of effectiveness, but is still considered safe. Specifically, for lithium this is a concentration in the blood of this drug of 0.5 to 1.5 milligrams per deciliter (mg/dl). At or below the lower level it is thought not to be effective. Above the higher level severe toxicity, resulting even in death, may occur. In my own experience I found that during the first four years of treatment I suffered from no manic episodes. Subsequently, there were many relapses of mania despite having the defined therapeutic blood concentration.

Lithium has many side effects. Among them are fetal toxicity, thyroid dysfunction (a thyroid-stimulating hormone level, TSH, should be measured in a blood test every six months), weight gain, tremor (shaking of the hands), increased urination and possibly kidney disease (renal function should be followed by checking serum creatinine levels, though this is not very sensitive). The thyroid abnormality induced by lithium can be readily correctable by prescribing thyroid hormone. Weight gain is disturbing to many and commonly associated with many of the drugs utilized in the treatment of bipolar disorder. The tremor is sometimes treated, with variable success, by prescribing a drug called a beta-blocker. As is the case in many of the situations encountered, the medication used to remedy one side effect carries with it another set of detrimental effects. Impotence is one of those observed with a beta-blocker. If renal injury develops, lithium should be discontinued. Side effects I personally experienced were thyroid malfunction (requiring treatment with thyroid hormone), tremor, and increased urination. Although my blood creatinine is normal, renal injury may have occurred. Initially I also developed dizziness, but this problem soon dissipated.

Valproic acid (the generic name), commonly known under its trade name Depakote, has more recently been approved by the FDA as a mood-stabilizing agent. Both names will be used interchangeably throughout this chapter. Prior to FDA approval for its use to treat manic depression, Depakote had been on the market to treat epilepsy and is thus termed an anticonvulsant. As for lithium, the mechanism of action of valproic acid remains unclear. Blood concentration levels are monitored to determine the amount to be taken to achieve a level that is considered primarily to be safe and secondly effective.

This range has been quantified as 50-100 mg/dl. However, as with lithium, I became manic despite having a concentration of valproic acid in this effective range. This occurred within less than six months after commencing use. Fetal toxicity has been described with Depakote use. Liver toxicity is another serious adverse effect of the drug and therefore liver enzymes need to be measured early when treatment is initiated and then monitored on at least a yearly basis. If these enzymes are elevated it may well be necessary to reduce (or possibly discontinue) the dose of Depakote. Hair loss is also a possible side effect of valproic acid. It should also be noted that using valproic acid can affect the levels of other drugs the patient may be taking.

Carbamazepine is an antiepileptic medication that had been used to treat bipolar disorder before Depakote. Though never FDA-approved for this use, it is still widely employed for mood stabilization. The mechanism for this drug is also unknown. For carbamazepine the therapeutic blood concentration is considered to be 7-11 mg/dl. Similar to my use of lithium and Depakote, I had relapses of mania despite this desired blood concentration. Manic episodes also occurred when both lithium and Tegretol were prescribed at the same time. Potential side effects of Tegretol use are bone marrow suppression resulting in reduced blood cell counts, liver damage, impaired coordination due to brain effects and dizziness or vertigo caused by uncontrollable eye movement. These side effects may be limited by reducing the dosage. The most significant side effect I encountered due to Tegretol was a dramatic case of vertigo. I could barely walk, let alone drive. With a slight reduction in dose the problem was resolved. As with Depakote, treatment with Tegretol can alter the concentrations of other medications and can cause fetal toxicity.

Several other antiepileptic drugs are now beginning to be employed either alone or as adjunctive therapy in manic depression. Gabapentin (Neurontin) and lamotrigene (Lamictal) are the most frequently used. Information on their effectiveness in bipolar disorder is scarce at this time. I have not been treated with either of these medications.

Antipsychotics

Examples of antipsychotic drugs are chlor-promazine (Thorazine) and haloperidol (Haldol). They tend to be sedating and rapid in action if injected. There can be numerous side effects. One class of these is called "autonomic" effects. These include a dry mouth from decreased saliva production, constipation and light-headedness, most prominently when attempting to stand. These are more prevalent with Throrazine. Another group of undesired consequences seen more frequently in other antipsychotics including Haldol are so-called Parkinsonian side effects, because they resemble or pro-duce the symptoms seen in Parkinson's dis-ease. These are also termed extrapyramidal symptoms, or EPS, and include tremors, stiff-ness and slow movement.

I have been administered Haldol on a few occasions. On most of these it clearly did not mitigate my manic psychosis. Conversely in others it may have had a beneficial effect. On the other hand, I did experience side effects. The Parkinsonian symptoms that developed included stiffness from my back to the tips of my fingers. However, these were insignificant compared to the akathisia, or "restless legs," Haldol also produced. I found this to be terribly uncomfortable, and I found only limited relief by continually walking. This compelling need to be pacing might be confused with the agitation or hyperactivity that is a symptom of the disease. The difference is that the severe walking associated with the disease will end, usually within 48 hours, whereas the drug-induced pacing will not stop unless the medication dose is lowered to the point of cessation.

A specific aim of the more recently developed antipsychotics was to minimize the severity of the side effects associated with older ones described previously. The new-generation of drugs are termed atypical antipsychotics and include risperidone (Risperdal), olanzapine (Zyprexa) and quetiapine fumarate (Seroquel). To counter some of these untoward effects of the antipsychotics of either the older or newer generation, psychiatrists often prescribe more medications that have no bearing on the primary disease of manic depression. These have side effects of their own and are not necessarily effective in mitigating the initial side effect(s) they were intended to relieve. Thus, the dose of antipsychotic prescribed usually proceeds along the following paradigm: Begin treatment with a standard dose. With the onset of significant side effects, secondary drugs will be added. If the side-effect symptoms remain intolerable, then another one of the medications may be substituted or possibly a reduction in dose of the initial antipsychotic will be attempted.

I have been prescribed each of these newer antipsychotics on separate occasions. Their effectiveness is unclear. Risperidone has very similar side effects to Haldol with Parkinsonian symptoms and akathisia. Seroquel was rather benign but was discontinued because at the time I was experiencing excessive fatigue and tiredness. Zyprexa was initiated in place of Seroquel, but Parkinsonian symptoms developed at the recommended dosage of 5 mg/day. These were not alleviated with secondary drugs such as benztropine (Cogentin) or amantadine. It was thus decided to reduce the dose to 2.5 mg/day, resulting in acceptable, though not complete, relief. One of the major drawbacks of the atypical antipsychotics is that they are far more expensive than the older drugs.

Antidepressants

There are a number of different types of antidepressants. Those most widely prescribed today are the selective serotonin reuptake inhibitors (SSRIs), including fluoxetine (Prozac), and the older tricyclic antidepressants (TCAs) and monoamine oxidase inhibitors (MAOs). Wellbutrin is another antidepressant but does not fall into any of the these categories. There is no existing theory of the mechanism of Wellbutrin in contrast to the other antidepressants that are considered to increase serotonin or both serotonin and norepinephrine neurotransmitter concentrations in the synaptic space. Many of these medications are employed for a number of other maladies from eating disorders to headaches to smoking cessation. These drugs usually require days to weeks to take effect.

Side effects with the SSRIs are considered relatively unlikely but include anxiety, decreased appetite and sexual dysfunction. The TCAs have deleterious consequences more frequently, that range from urinary symptoms to potentially lethal heart rhythm abnormalities. The MAOs can be toxic when the patient consumes wine or cheese. Of significant importance in treating manic depression is the possibility of triggering mania, especially when the person has only experienced a depression(s) and has yet to be diagnosed as having bipolar disorder. Therefore antidepressants are usually avoided in a patient with confirmed bipolar disorder. However if the depression is severe, Wellbutrin is considered to have the least risk of precipitating mania. It is cautioned that Wellbutrin not be administered to an individual with a history of seizures.

On more than one occasion following the resolution of my manic symptoms, I developed intense depressions to the extent I was near comatose. It was deemed necessary to reverse this situation, in part, with the aid of an antidepressant. Wellbutrin was chosen because of its aforementioned low risk of producing a relapse of mania. Whether Wellbutrin had any positive effect I cannot be certain, but I did not have any discernable side effects.

General Considerations

As discussed earlier, effectiveness of medications in treating a behavioral disorder is difficult to assess largely due to the subjective interpretation of behavior. The difficulty is manifested in how investigators define success. How severe have been the mood swings before the treatment fails? Few of the drugs discussed have ever gone beyond one-year trials. How long must one go without a manic event to say it is successful? Furthermore, often the side-effects of medications are not emphasized, as I have found with respect to my treatment with Haldol and the subsequent onset of akathisia. This is a common side effect, but it was not taken into account by my psychiatrists. I have also experienced cognitive impairment with lithium use. Once again, this extremely important side effect was not discussed with me prior to treatment.

The FDA determines which medications may be lawfully sold in this country. It must be satisfied that the drug is both safe and efficacious in treating at least one disorder. Needless to say, this is a difficult task because serious adverse effects may not appear for years or develop in the next generation. Political forces unquestionably are involved in the evaluation process. Doctors and patients may pressure for approval of a drug that is legal in another country or, likewise, make a decision based on promising available research studies. Similarly, pharmaceutical companies may lobby in order to profit from their investment. An important point to understand is that once approved for a specific disease, the medication can then be prescribed for other conditions as well — this is called an "off-label" use of the drug. This frequently occurs because it is costly to obtain approval for each use.

If medications are legally available, there are several different situations that must be considered in regard to their implementation. The primary caveat involving the use of any drug is that it is dispensed with the objective that the improvement in the course or symptoms of the disease exceeds the toxic side effects or other adverse consequences of its use. Looking at the pharmacological treatment of various medical conditions can provide some insight and be instructive as to how drug therapies should be instituted with respect to manic depression.

In general, medications are prescribed for either acute or chronic treatment of illnesses. With some medications in certain situations there is no alternative but to administer the agent, since it offers the only apparent hope of forestalling imminent death. This is exemplified when antibiotics are employed to cure an otherwise lethal infectious disease. They are administered despite some potential serious toxic effects such as kidney failure, hearing loss or life-threatening immunological reaction until the infection has resolved. Although not necessarily as clear, the disturbed thought processes in mania accompanied by the highly agitated energetic state may require immediate treatment to avoid likely death from suicide or as a consequence of other dangerous behavior (reckless driving, illicit drug use, etc.). The drugs used to alleviate the psychosis rarely have lethal side effects.

For other disease states pharmacological agents are used on an acute basis, not to avoid death, but rather to lessen the severity of symptoms until these agents are no longer necessary. An example of these drugs would be narcotic pain medications prescribed after surgery or injuries. As most people realize with narcotics, there is the potential for developing an addiction among other undesirable effects such as altered thoughts. But the temporary relief of severe pain takes high priority, and thus the medication treatment is implemented. In manic depression tranquiliz-ing medications such as diazepam (Valium) may be employed temporarily to help sedate a manic individual. A small risk of addiction accompanies use of this class of drugs.

Chronic, incurable diseases often require medications to be used on a long-term basis to sustain the life of the patient. A prime illustration is Type I diabetes mellitus, where the patient must inject insulin daily to survive. Insulin is a hormone secreted by the pan-creas. Its prime function is the regulation of blood glucose levels. Despite existing natu-rally in the human body, it must be adminis-tered with care. For example, imminent death can occur if excess insulin is injected (hypoglycemic shock). The dose of insulin depends on blood-sugar concentrations. Thyroid abnormalities are frequently associat-ed with bipolar disorder. The thyroid gland secretes thyroid hormone into the blood that then affects metabolism throughout the body. If the thyroid gland is inactive, thyroid hormone must be taken daily as replacement therapy to ensure that all of these metabolic processes continue in a normal manner. Similar to insulin, this is a natural compound produced by the body. And similarly the correct dose must be taken to avoid severe injury. This dose can be precisely ascertained by checking blood levels of the pituitary hormone referred to previously, TSH.

Elevated cholesterol is another chronic condition treated frequently with medication. In this instance the cholesterol-lowering agent has no immediate (if any) impact on reversing arterial plaque buildup, and therefore reducing cholesterol may not be efficacious in warding off future cardiac disease. However, the data collected are rather convincing that these medications do reduce the incidence of heart attacks and that the side effects are minimal, but on rare occasions can be serious. Some individuals will not respond to the medication (cholesterol levels are not reduced) and thus there is no reason to continue treatment. Even if the drug does lower cholesterol, the treatment may not be commenced because the price of these medications can be substantial, or the patient may find it inconvenient to follow the daily regimen. In manic depression the disease is serious enough in most instances that lifetime prophylactic medication treatment with mood stabilizers is mandatory. Unfortunately, the only means to monitor effectiveness is by assessing behavior without having an additional, more objective parameter such as a blood chemical level.

In all of these instances it is important that the patient be educated and be knowledgeable about why the drug is prescribed. Then he should be aware of what the potential risks and benefits associated with using it are. Finally, after consultation with the physician, the patient should (in most cases) render the final decision about whether or not to commence therapy with the medicine. This will engender an alliance with the physician. More importantly, the educated patient who is an active participant in the pharmacological management of his illness will most likely adhere to the medical treatment regimen and have an enhanced probability of favorable response. Sometimes this discussion with the patient is difficult or impossible, such as when the patient's brain is incapacitated, and therefore the family or the physician may have the responsibility of deciding if medication therapy should be implemented. A patient suffering from manic depression may be irrational and therefore require medication in an attempt to best ensure his safety and to help him regain normal thought. As a final note, even when pharmacologic therapy appears effective, family support must be at least equally emphasized not only as treatment but to provide ever-vigilant close observation of the patient, because there will almost always remain a risk of future manic, as well as depressive, episodes.

chapter four:

how is manic depression treated?

---

1. How is manic depression treated?

Stan: Manic depression cannot be cured and can be difficult to control. As I described in Chapter 2 about my own experience, treatment usually begins when the patient is symptomatic in the first acute manic episode. Medical care is initiated at this time because it is only after the patient's expansive behavior is dramatically disruptive and/or he is in distress that the illness is usually diagnosed. This first encounter with the psychiatric health care system is vastly different from the chronic control of the disease. Without continuing treatment, the patient has a significant risk of deterioration of behavior eventually resulting in a total disruption of normal life or even death.

Even if depressions precede the manic episode, for several reasons medical treatment is often not started until the manic breakthrough. First, there is a stigma attached to psychiatric care. Second, people do not realize that manic depression is a physical disease of the brain that can potentially be treated. Last, depressive episodes are usually less conspicuous than manic ones. The failure to seek treatment is extremely unfortunate since lives can be irreparably harmed due to the melancholic state. Failure in school or work, personal relationships (e.g., divorce) and even suicide are common consequences. One important cautionary note documented in the psychiatric journals is that treatment with antidepressant medications can stimulate a patient with bipolar disorder into mania.

Acute mania is a psychiatric emergency. As such it is critical to get the patient out of the community and into a "safe" environment as the first step of treatment. The resident physician made me aware of the term "safe" during my first hospitalization. He did not define it at that time and I have not heard it used since then even though safety is a critical part of any treatment. My first hospitalization occurred after I was picked up at the airport by security guards. It is typically the case that the first hospitalization is involuntary. Often it is the task of the family to have a patient committed. Therefore, it is imperative to understand how and why a patient should be made safe. The process of committing a loved one to a psychiatric ward is a dreadful experience for both the patient and his family. The manic person will often disdain the concern of loved ones and may flee to avoid the loss of freedom incurred by hospitalization.

A safe environment is one that will prevent the patient from unwittingly breaking the law. Rarely are patients in acute mania violent, but they may need to be protected from others who misunderstand manic behavior, and thus inappropriately feel threatened by it. The safe environment also prevents the individual from driving, because he may be reckless, and prevents travel, for this desire is often delusional. Such travel is one manifestation of the buying-spree behavior that can cause financial ruin. Furthermore, the safe environment should restrict a patient's access to all finances and so help him avoid squandering savings or doing damage to credit ratings. Safety also includes restricted phone access because through this outlet the patient can interact with society much as if he were on the street. This is true for any other communication technology, most notably the Internet. I cannot emphasize too much the importance of early placement in a safe haven to help the patient avoid the dire consequences of this disease, which include loss of employment, damage to relationships or death from acting on delusions (e.g., jumping off a building to fly). These consequences can provide motivation, albeit a negative one, for loved ones to overcome the difficulties associated with maintaining a safe environment.

The safe environment is usually a hospital, but outpatient care with a loved one at home is more desirable if safety can be maintained. However, if the patient is to be safe outside the hospital he must be compliant.

Another possible safe environment is jail. Many manic patients are put in jail because of their erratic and disruptive behavior. In some ways this is better than being on the streets. However, although the patient is removed from society while in jail, further medical care is unlikely to ensue there, and a criminal record may result. Additionally, to state the obvious, jail is inherently more dangerous than a hospital because of the violent tendencies of some of the inmates.

I experienced several techniques that were helpful when I was hospitalized. Dim lighting, reduced interaction with other patients, even being kept in isolation reduced stimulation of my mania. Unfortunately on several occasions, isolation and the use of physical constraints were simply used for the convenience of hospital personnel. This might seem to be barbaric, inhumane treatment. However, I realize that Mr. Hyde can appear to behave almost like a monster that requires extreme physical measures to subdue him. Furthermore, to be fair, the hospital staff usually had a large number of patients to deal with and were unaware of my nonviolent nature.

With the patient in a safe environment, the psychiatrist can perform the steps described in Chapter 2 toward formulating a diagnosis. Treatment can begin once a preliminary diagnosis of manic depression is established. An antipsychotic may initially be necessary to break the mania. If the individual will not cooperate and voluntarily take the medication, or if quicker action is desired, intramuscular injection may be the method of delivery rather than a pill. If the patient's energy and loss of reality persist, repeated administration of the antipsychotic medication may be required. Administration of a benzodiazepine class of drugs (Valium is the most recognized of these) may also be considered, orally or by injection, to sedate the energetic, uncontrolled person.

When the patient is stabilized to the point of complying with medication, treatment with a mood stabilizer is usually started. Up until the last few years, lithium would have been the drug of choice. Now valproic acid (Depakote) is also considered to be effective. Other agents of the anticonvulsant class are also available but generally not used on an initial basis. None of these medications can be administered by injection and therefore some control is necessary to begin their use. The concentration of these medications in the bloodstream must be established to obtain a therapeutic level and to prevent toxicity. Lithium must be monitored very carefully because it can become severely toxic and possibly lethal even at low levels. To avoid gastrointestinal effects (nausea, diarrhea, stomach upset, etc.) the anticonvulsants usually are started at a low dose and then increased incrementally until a therapeutic blood level is attained. I should emphasize that unlike the antipsychotic and benzodiazepine agents that exert their effects rapidly (within minutes to hours), the effects of these mood-stabilizing drugs may not begin to appear for two weeks or more. A more detailed discussion on the pharmacology of manic depression is located in Chapter 3.

Few long-term studies are available, but most psychiatrists believe that without the continued use of medications symptoms of the illness will increase in frequency and intensity. The chronic medical treatment of this disorder usually consists of one or more mood stabilizers, possibly an antipsychotic and the continued use of a benzodiazepine. Whether environmental modification, including insights from the patient himself, can have a significant effect on the course of the illness has not yet been documented.

I have found from personal experience that stress reduction, awareness of the nature of the disease and maintaining optimism are helpful in controlling the illness.

Admittedly, these are not always easily achieved. For example, the financial ruin induced by the disease may result in severe stress. If left unchecked, symptoms, most notably of mania but also of depression, can be amplified, impairing the patient's awareness of the state of the illness. Similarly, the very nature of the depressions will directly dim the patient's optimism and contribute to worsening the patient's condition. The family support system becomes vital for providing objective awareness and other aspects of the environmental care for this disease. I discovered most painfully that I could not depend on the professional medical system for this support. Other networks, such as support groups and coworkers, were also incapable of fulfilling this function.

For an individual experiencing a major depressive episode, the ultimate danger is suicide. The hospital is accepted as a place of safety for a patient where "suicide precautions" can be employed. However, even these precautions are not always effective, for suicides do occur within hospitals. These preventive measures had been instituted for me on one occasion, namely locking me in a totally empty room without my clothes. If anything, this treatment reduced my desire to live. It is therefore arguable whether hospitalization actually saves lives from this fatal act. Even if suicide is prevented during the hospitalization, the stay may be as short as two days and this may be only a minor postponement. What I am stating here is an example where what is accepted is often not the reality, i.e., that the safe environment of the hospital does not fulfill its function.

It is critical that physicians be especially cautious when administering an antidepressant to a depressed individual with even a mild case of bipolar disorder. Antidepressants have been documented in the psychiatric literature as having the capability of precipitating a manic episode. Fortunately, the medications have been refined over the course of many years and now have fewer side effects than in the past. The duration of treatment with medications for depression has not been clearly specified. Similar to the mood stabilizers for mania, a patient who is undergoing a major depressive episode may not feel the mood-elevating effects of the medication for weeks. Psychotherapy that verbally makes the patient aware of his impaired view of the world and allows him to explore the causes of possible underlying depression-inducing circumstances is necessary. This is best accomplished by family who have the personal knowledge and time to be effective.

As alluded to earlier, modification of the patient's lifestyle to reduce environmental stressors that may incite symptoms should be seriously considered. In fact, this aspect of care might be as critical as medication for maintaining long-term health. In my case, I eventually determined that my illness could not be controlled while I was enrolled in a medical residency program. Of course, in a sense this was an admission of a partial victory for the illness because my life's goals were altered.

I have presented the basics of treatment. Without a doubt, a safe environment is the first priority whether it be at home or in a hospital. Medication should then be instituted after a preliminary diagnosis is determined. This diagnosis depends on the physician obtaining information about the patient's past personality. Once stability is obtained, chronic medication generally ensues. Vital to treatment at this stage is a knowledgeable support system that provides an environment conducive to minimizing mood variability.

Ira: I will answer this question in a much more general manner than Stan by categorizing the treatment of manic depression into three broad areas. First, the illness must be diagnosed, as described in Chapter 2. Second, a long-term regime of medication and observation must be put in place. And third, during periods of acute mania, the patient must be brought under control and into safety. I will describe in a following question that the delegation of responsibility among medical professionals and the family will have a profound effect on the patient's well-being.

2. Why don't regular doctors treat manic depression?

Stan: The thrust of this question concerns the isolation of manic depression to the domain of psychiatry despite its organic origin. Most physicians do not treat manic depression for a number of reasons. Due to the specialization prevalent in medicine today, physicians are not adequately trained in this area, usually spending no more than two months during medical school on mental illnesses and psychiatry. Furthermore, as in most fields, the pace of change related to the treatment of manic depression makes keeping abreast difficult for non-specialists. The difficulty and time demands of treating this illness also discourage physicians who are not psychiatrists from addressing this illness.

Ira: Traditionally psychiatrists have treated mental disorders, and so they continue to do so. I also believe that of all physicians, they are the only ones who are trained to talk to patients. This is a critical tool in treating manic depression. However, no physicians, even psychiatrists, are trained to talk to families. This important shortcoming in training will be discussed as part of the following question.

3. What do psychiatrists do?

Stan: A psychiatrist is a medical doctor, thus he has graduated from a four-year college and four years of medical school. Four more years of training are required after medical school, including a small amount (six months) of training in general medicine. The psychiatrist then takes an exam that, if passed, confers upon him the title of Diplomat of the American Board of Psychiatry and Neurology. The neurology designation is misleading because psychiatrists typically have little knowledge of or experience with neurology. A psychologist is sometimes confused with a psychiatrist. A psychologist has not graduated from medical school and is therefore not an M.D, but is still called "doctor" because he has completed a Ph.D. A clinical psychologist interviews and tests patients for the purpose of diagnosis and/or providing psychotherapy, but is prohibited from prescribing medications.

In the typical doctor-patient relationship, the doctor attempts to solve a problem by the request of the patient. On the other hand, a manic depression patient may not be aware of a problem and the psychiatrist sees him only as the result of the concern or insistence of others (family, friends, coworkers, a physician in a different specialty or the police). Regardless of the patient's condition, the psychiatrist must get an adequate history of the patient's behavior. However, the patient in either the elevated or depressed state may be unable to provide an objective or complete explanation of the circumstances of his problem that resulted in his being examined. Neither the textbooks that psychiatry residents study nor their clinical training emphasize the importance of seeking information from a source other than the patient. Our experience has clearly demonstrated that psychiatrists do not seek out this information from others. Ira has made himself available to discuss my situation time and time again, yet he has rarely been consulted. This has been unfortunate because my care and life have definitely suffered as a result. On one occasion I was actually discharged from the hospital without my family being notified while I was still in the manic state.

In regard to diagnosis, to no significant extent do psychiatrists explicitly employ the criteria defined in the *DSM-IV*. Among the possible reasons for this are poor training, insufficient time and resources, lazy practices or lack of a belief in the *DSM-IV*.

There are two fundamental approaches to treating manic depression. The first, which is oriented toward psychotherapy, stresses the behavioral approach to treatment, because it is assumed that mental illnesses are learned from or molded by the environment and can be modified by instruction or other external influences. The second paradigm is the pharmacological approach. This is the typical model in the current practice, where the assumption of manic depression being a physical malfunction indicates that medication is the proper mode of treatment. Manic depression is not thought to respond well to "talk" therapy by psychiatrists who use the pharmacological approach. Indeed, most psychiatrists prescribe medication as their sole treatment. This neglects the "talk" therapy that is required to evaluate the efficacy of the medication. Furthermore, psychiatrists do not discuss the patient's condition with the family even though in many, if not most, instances the family can provide better information about the progress of the patient than the patient can himself. This situation has contributed to the many failures of my medication to prevent manic episodes.

In the limited time the psychiatrist does interact with the patient, he can gather direct information about his state of mind and function from his appearance ("body language") and speech. The astute clinician is keenly aware of both of these during the office visit, especially the latter. Besides providing insight into the patient's condition, such visits can also build an important alliance that may aid in treating the disorder during a future manic episode.

I should now give a word of caution about the capability of the psychiatrist. The uncertainty that surrounds many of the environmental influences and the inability to specify the physical abnormality leave the psychiatrist in a very compromised position. It is clear to me as both an electrical engineer who has experience with human-designed systems and a physician and physiologist knowledgeable about biological systems (pulmonary, cardiac, renal, endocrine, etc.), that there is relatively little understanding of the central nervous system. This has led me to conclude that the psychiatrist is in the unenviable position of minimally understanding the mechanisms of the illness he is attempting to treat.

Ira: Stan has described the basic functions of the psychiatrist. I will describe what psychiatrists cannot do and what I think they should do, because it is important for the expectations of patients and families to coincide with reality.

Physicians have an exalted place in our society. When we are sick we put ourselves completely in their hands. They are equipped with high-tech instruments that give them information about the fundamental processes of life. Not only are we passive subjects under their direction, but we expect them to be highly knowledgeable beyond our understanding, and to effectively cure us. Perhaps this description of modern medicine is simplistic, but it is important that patients and families develop much lower expectations for the care provided by psychiatrists for the treatment of manic depression. In fact, I would describe the care of manic depression by psychiatrists as *impotent* beyond giving advice about and prescribing medications.

It took me many years of observing the performance of many psychiatrists to come to this conclusion. I do not fault them for their impotence, but they should recognize it and relate their capabilities and inabilities honestly to their patients and families. I am no longer frustrated by their impotence because I understand it and recognize that it derives from the very nature of the illness and the way psychiatrists must do their jobs. Thus, it would be like being frustrated with gravity for not allowing me to float wherever I desired. That is, to be frustrated and angry about the fundamental nature of something is self-defeating and foolish.

Consider the three broad areas required for treatment that I described in question 1 (diagnosis, long-term care, care during acute mania) as they relate to the capabilities of psychiatrists. I said in Chapter 2 that changes in personality or mood are a key to diagnosis. But invariably, the psychiatrist becomes acquainted with the patient only after symptoms have become obvious to others. It is highly unlikely that the psychiatrist will have any baseline knowledge of the patient's personality. In Stan's case it was only after being picked up and transported to the hospital by airport security that medication was initiated. His previous visits to the psychiatrist resulted in no actual treatment prior to the catastrophic event of his initial hospitalization. In effect, this is like having a heart attack after a visit to a cardiologist where no treatment was initiated.

In long-term care the psychiatrist prescribes prophylactic medication and meets with the patient on a regular basis to judge its effectiveness. Without exception, psychiatrists have been unable to make this judgement adequately during Stan's extended treatment. For example, on one visit to his psychiatrist on which I accompanied him, the doctor confided to me in private how well Stan was doing. I had to inform her that at that moment Stan was manic to the point that he believed himself to be God. This psychiatrist was on the faculty of a teaching hospital that has one of the leading research programs on manic depression.

During an acute manic episode psychiatrists have a severely limited capacity to assist in delivering a patient safely to treatment. On only one occasion has Stan's psychiatrist attempted to assist me in getting Stan to the hospital. It turned out he was no help whatsoever, and it was only due to his inexperience that he even made the effort. On another occasion I called a different psychiatrist long distance to inform him Stan was manic and needed hospitalization. Stan was scheduled to see him that day and he even went to his office. But he did not prevent Stan from leaving his office to start a manic spending spree that would take him from his home in Kentucky to the island of Kauai in Hawaii.

The basis of the impotence I have described stems from the limited time a psychiatrist can spend with any particular patient. It is typical for a patient to meet with his psychiatrist for one half-hour per month in the absence of manic symptoms. While not in the hospital, the greatest frequency with which Stan has seen his psychiatrist is once per week, with the exception of each weekday for a short period after one manic episode. Yet comprehending a personality for the purpose of diagnosis and long-term treatment would require that the psychiatrist essentially be on continuous call for an individual patient. This would not only be limited to an acute manic episode but would involve the near full-time personal support required during the post-manic period as well. This is impossible for any psychiatrist, for he has many patients, not to mention a personal life of his own.

But psychiatrists are not totally ineffective. I would suggest they can provide the following critical services that derive from their training and experience, qualities usually lacking in family members who must provide the bulk of the care.

1. A psychiatrist must perform the key function of diagnosis.
2. The psychiatrist should understand and employ knowledge of physiology, pharmacology and psychology or talk therapy in treatment.
3. The psychiatrist should assist the patient and family with the social implications of the disease, especially legal issues. This

topic will be addressed in the following chapters.

4. The psychiatrist should pay close attention to and direct logistics, especially making arrangements for hospitalization.

Bringing a manic patient to the emergency room without prior notice is a harrowing experience. It is especially frustrating when a psychiatrist was supposed to have made arrangements. Unfortunately, this has been a common occurrence in my experience. For example, in one case I had arranged with Stan's psychiatrist to move him from one hospital to another. He was to arrange for his admission. However, nothing had been arranged and Stan was not cooperative. I spent several difficult hours in the emergency room. I was finally able to contact the psychiatrist. When I explained the situation, he made a joke about it and then hung up on me.

When performing the functions listed above, the psychiatrist must be keenly aware that the knowledge and tools for treating mental illness are limited. That is, the psychiatrist should understand his fundamental impotence and thus perform his functions with humility. This humility will allow the psychiatrist to perform his most important function: to initially and regularly enlist, encourage and educate the patient and family, making them full partners in, if not leaders of, the treatment team.

4. How do you pick a psychiatrist?

Stan: Choosing a psychiatrist to treat bipolar disorder is similar to choosing a physician to treat other illnesses: one looks at their qualifications, training and recommendations. However, as discussed in the previous question, the psychiatrist's cooperation and collaboration with the patient and family are absolutely critical in the treatment of manic depression. I believe making sure that a psychiatrist understands this most important issue is the key to picking a psychiatrist. The initial interview should occur with the family present. A patient should be sensitive to how the psychiatrist discusses treatment with him: determine if he talks with him or to him.   There are also several specific issues related to choosing a psychiatrist.

Confidentiality in the doctor-patient relationship is important for all branches of medicine but is especially so with regard to psychiatry. But what may seem contradictory is that what is discussed with the psychiatrist must be confidential in general but not with regard to the designated support system. This point is a key message of this book.

Treating an illness such as manic depression requires that the psychiatrist perceive changes in personality. Furthermore, because the illness affects every aspect of life, personal matters will have a direct bearing on treatment. Thus, it would be very helpful if the psychiatrist in some sense could be considered a friend who has a genuine interest in a patient's life and how it is progressing. Furthermore, the psychiatrist should offer to assist in life matters where reasonable. For example, he should give advice and assistance on disability issues, employment, how to handle questions related to the disease in social situations, etc. In short, choose a psychiatrist who would take note of the patient as a person, not only as a patient.

Ira: In the previous question I have described what psychiatrists are capable of doing, and thus what they should be doing. During the first meeting with a psychiatrist the patient and family should discuss these recommendations about family involvement with the psychiatrist. However, I have come to have so little regard for the capabilities of psychiatrists in general that I believe the role of the psychiatrist in Stan's care is inconsequential beyond writing prescriptions for medications. I realize that this is a strong statement, but it is a fact.

5. What role does a therapist or counselor have in treatment?

Stan: A therapist or counselor is sometimes used to perform some of the non-medical tasks we have described for psychiatrists. A therapist was enlisted for my treatment on one occasion. In my treatment schedule I saw the psychiatrist once a month and the therapist weekly. The psychiatrist would primarily handle any medication issues and briefly ask me how I was doing. The therapist, who worked in the same office as the psychiatrist, would delve deeper into my life situations in hourly sessions. We believed that these medical professionals together could manage my illness better than a psychiatrist could alone. This was a miscalculation, however, because this system of treatment eventually failed. After four months in Tennessee under their care I became acutely manic. The therapist saw me in this condition during a routinely scheduled session. She recognized that I had destabilized and, on her own initiative, called a nearby pharmacy to prescribe an antipsychotic (denying my illness, of course, I never picked it up) without consulting the psychiatrist. I would have hoped she would have contacted the psychiatrist, who could have then had me admitted to the hospital. Instead, I was allowed to leave the office in a manic state. Eventually, Ira became aware of the reappearance of Mr. Hyde and was forced to fly to Nashville from Durham to take me to the hospital. In essence, through this and other experiences, we came realize that there is no substitute for the family as the support system in handling this illness. Even the most dedicated therapist cannot devote the time and attention required. This does not eliminate the therapist's possible contribution, but patients and families must realize such treatment is limited and that there must be extensive communication between the family and the psychiatrist about the patient's condition. As a final note, I was so disturbed by the therapist's response to my relapse that I refused to see her again and stated this in no uncertain terms to my psychiatrist.

6. What has been your experience with mental hospitals?

Stan: There are three different categories of hospitals that treat psychiatric patients: private hospitals, university hospitals and state or public institutions (including veterans' hospitals). The private hospitals are either regular hospitals that have a ward specifically for psychiatric patients or hospitals dedicated only to treatment of the mentally ill. The patients are usually controlled and stable, and are rarely acutely manic. The age range is broad and distributed in an equal manner on the adult wards, ranging from about 20 to 65, with equal numbers of men and women. There is often a kitchenette on the ward and a day room. The rooms are usually private with a bathroom and otherwise bland but clean with a bed and dresser the only furniture. It is only in the past few decades that mentally ill people have been allowed to stay in community facilities; formerly they were hospitalized only in asylums removed from the populace.

University hospitals usually offer patients state-of-the-art care. This is because they are teaching hospitals with some of the faculty active in research. But the medications prescribed and treatment regimens for manic depression actually differ very little among the various types of hospitals. In a university hospital the physician is usually a resident and/or a medical student and there is only peripheral contact with the attending faculty member.

State institutions usually treat those patients who have no insurance or require more physical restraint than is typically available at the other hospitals. The patients here were usually younger, with a mean age in the early 20's with equal sex ratio, though the wards were not always coed as in the hospitals discussed above. A greater number of patients tended to be much more ill and required prolonged inpatient care. The physicians were often of foreign origin at the state institutions but generally more concerned with the well-being of the patients. This was true even though the patient-to-physician ratio, and thus the workload, was greater. I never found culture differences to be a barrier in communication with the foreign-born psychiatrists. I believe genuine concern surpasses such boundaries. The staff at most of the state hospitals also functioned differently from those at the other types. They demonstrated a greater concern and interest in the patients. Corresponding to the sincerity of the physicians and staff, I noticed more improvement in the mental health of this population. The fact that they were sicker in the first place may also have contributed to this.

The benefits of private hospitals over the state facilities are that they are generally much newer, cleaner, quieter with private rooms and have more choice of foods. The state hospital usually did not offer any snacks between the three main meals. The state hospitals recognized the importance of exercise more than the other hospitals. This may have also reflected the younger age and longer hospital stays of the patients. Some patients in the state institutions would be more ill and potentially dangerous-mainly because of fighting.

I have described that the function of a mental hospital or the psychiatric wing of a regular hospital is to provide a safe environment and initiate treatment during acute mania and, to a lesser extent, during depression. In my experience they have performed this function adequately but with some significant failures, which I describe below. Similar to the treatment of other illnesses in a general hospital, the overall atmosphere and level of care at a mental hospital affect recovery from mania. Therefore I will also discuss these aspects of my stays at the various hospitals at which I was treated.

With regard to initiating treatment, in one instance while hospitalized with mania, I refused to take medications but no effort was made to force or persuade me to do so throughout my four-week stay. I was then transferred to another facility where, with a little negotiation, the physician convinced me to begin treatment. There were two other occasions during which I expressed displeasure about taking medication because of my manic thoughts, but in both instances a short explanation by an obviously concerned and caring physician convinced me to comply. Thus, I believe it is important at every level to make the effort to communicate with a manic patient.

In terms of providing a safe environment to protect me from my mania, hospitals failed me on two occasions. In my second hospitalization I was admitted to the private community hospital. Part of the standard protocol in the process of rehabilitation there was to allow patients to spend some time away from the hospital on a pass in order to facilitate reintegration into normal life activities on a limited basis. Following a week in the hospital, I was given a pass. When I arrived home I became impulsive and uncontrolled. I first discarded the keyboard, mouse and a new modem for my computer. Then for no reason I called one of my female colleagues where I was training. This disturbed and possibly frightened (though there was no direct suggestion of violence) this individual, as Mr. Hyde frequently does. Ira was subsequently notified of this impaired social behavior and acted swiftly to return me to the hospital well before the allotted time. A few days later I was discharged without my family's knowledge and another hospitalization ensued shortly thereafter because I was actually still manic.

Another failure at maintaining a safe environment occurred at an academic hospital. I was allowed to make innumerable, successive, scatological phone calls to Ira's house impulsively and irrationally. I also made rapid, repeated telephone calls long distance to the hospital where I was completing my residency training. I did not use obscene language during these calls but did speak with a tone of hostility. These calls were a contributing factor to my eventual dismissal.

Hospitalization for a psychiatric condition differs from that of physical illnesses in important ways. The patients frequently have much greater reservations about, if not outright indignation at, being there. This is starkly evident when there is a strong denial of the illness. Another difference with respect to medical ailments is that psychiatric hospitalization carries an enormous stigma and, thus, the patient receives less social support. The paucity of visitors and get-well cards for the patients reflects this as well. The combination of these factors may impair recovery that might otherwise be expected in these facilities. Another factor that I would like to mention is the lack of cleanliness particular to some of the old state psychiatric hospitals that made me very uncomfortable.

When I was a patient my typical day was uneventful in any of the types of psychiatric hospitals. The day revolved around the three meals that were served either in a cafeteria or on the ward. When there was an off-ward dining room, only stable patients were permitted to leave for eating purposes. Blood draws for analysis were done in the early morning prior to breakfast. Along with meals, medication dispensing was on a strict schedule. The remainder of the time was loosely organized at most of the facilities. This gave me the opportunity for contemplation or to talk to other patients. Television was usually available, but only in the communal day room, and there were some restrictions to when the patients could watch. Newspapers were not readily available. Some of the hospitals had group discussions on a broad range of topics such as medications, current events, meditation, arts and crafts, cooking, assertiveness training and on-site gardening. These were usually tedious to me because they were presented at a low intellectual level, but the other patients didn't show interest either.

The lifestyle in the state hospitals differed from the others in that it had a regimented tone similar to that of a military organization with inspections twice per day and a strong presence of authority. In fact, one of the hospitals where I stayed was a former army base at which many of the employees were veterans. The patients were required to perform certain tasks such as making their beds and keeping their belongings organized. There were even inspections to check on compliance of these tasks. It should be emphasized that the patients there required this type of authority because of their young age, and, to a lesser extent, because of their mental illnesses.

Ira: We have described why achieving safety for the patient is critical during an acute manic episode. Of course the hospital plays a key role in accomplishing this goal. It is out of fashion now to call a mental hospital an insane asylum but the word asylum is apt, given that an asylum is a sanctuary or refuge.

It was always a relief for me to get Stan into the hospital, but it was with mixed feelings. The hospital is effective because there it is possible to use physical force to subdue Mr. Hyde. But even when Hyde controlled Stan's body, it was difficult to witness him manhandled. This was especially the case when Stan was forcibly medicated.

Unfortunately, in our experience hospitals have not always fulfilled their primary function of keeping Stan safe. While being treated at one of the country's leading teaching hospitals Stan, as Mr. Hyde, was allowed to make scores of scatological phone calls. He also threw his wallet and contact lenses in the trash. For $650/day one would have thought the staff could have at least controlled this harmful behavior. The excuse I was given is that the law did not allow them to restrict his actions. In another instance recounted by Stan, he was released from the hospital while manic, and the hospital did not even attempt to inform us.

The incidents described here were at private hospitals. However, it is more than likely that eventually a manic patient will need to be placed in a public mental hospital because most insurance policies have inadequate coverage. The problem with public hospitals, and to a lesser degree private hospitals, is getting the patient admitted and keeping him there long enough until self-awareness of the illness has returned. A major factor related to this problem is that the patient usually wants to be released as soon as possible. As far as the hospital is concerned, the source of difficulty is certainly found in the law and in the way psychiatrists and other professionals perceive the law. This was the case discussed above, when Stan was allowed to undertake unsafe behavior while in the hospital. We shall discuss the law and mental illness in Chapter 8.

In addition, there is a general public ambivalence, which is reflected in the government, towards the treatment of mental illness, especially in terms of restricting the freedom of patients in mental wards. Perhaps this ambivalence was most popularly expressed in Ken Kesey's novel, and the subsequent movie, *One Flew Over the Cuckoo's Nest.* The social commentator Norman Podhoretz has explained this frame of mind as an offshoot of what he calls the *cult of authenticity.* While this view has been a long-term feature of American culture, it became predominant in the 60's in the form of a rejection of middle-class morals and manners. As Podhoretz explains, "And thus-in perhaps the most outlandish expression of this ethos, espoused by psychiatrists like R. D. Lang, poets like Allen Ginsberg, and novelists like Ken Kesey-schizophrenics and other sufferers from mental disease were more authentic human beings than those who had purchased a reputation for normality by conforming to the standards of a society that was itself truly insane."

The ultimate result of this ethos is a pervasive reluctance to restrict a patient's freedom, even among mental health professionals. This has also been reflected in a general release of patients from mental institutions and a decrease in funding for their maintenance. In some localities there is a severe shortage of mental wards as we found to our anguish in Nashville, TN. This tale is also reported in Chapter 8.

7. Are mental hospitals dangerous?

Stan: Some of the state hospitals that I was admitted to had patients who had violent tendencies. I surmised that these individuals were those who were young and physically healthy but had paranoid schizophrenia. I don't believe that they were fully aware of their destructive tendencies and actions. They did not have nearly as much pent-up anger as I noticed in individuals in jail, who clearly had a more significant propensity to be violent. I never had any serious confrontation in any of the psychiatric institutions, nor did any others that I noticed. However, I am aware that some of those who were uncontrolled were taken to a special ward. In contrast, one inmate was nearly killed in a vicious fight in my one stay in jail. Nonetheless, even in jail I was impressed with the demeanor of most of the inmates-at least in the cell in which I was confined, which was partially reserved for those with medical needs.

Although, and most critically, no medical attention was administered, in one sense the jail was better for my health because smoking was not permitted. Psychiatric patients in the state hospitals are notoriously profligate smokers, and one of the hospitals allowed this habit indoors, which I found personally noxious. I am confident that the restriction of freedom employed to create the safe environment is a factor that contributes to the urge to smoke. I was pleased the jail had a gym, though the inmates tended to purposely and subconsciously vent their anger and frustration on the basketball court. I made certain that I did not play where I would endanger myself by being too aggressive. At times this meant not participating because I knew my mere presence on the court was not safe.

8. How do medications help you?

Stan: It is very likely that the medications have some effectiveness, in some people, in alleviating some of the symptoms of this devastating disease. I discussed these drugs in detail in the essay on pharmacology (Chapter 3). However, I recognize that there is no absolute proof that this is true. Published studies and theories may be totally inaccurate because of the inherent uncertainty in measuring behavior and the "placebo effect."

In contrast to the uncertain benefit, I know that these drugs can cause physical harm and that this fact must be considered when a patient and his family are deciding whether and how to implement them. These concerns include dosages and duration of use of the medication. The prescription of more drugs to rectify, or at least mitigate, the side effects produced by the primary medications can result in even more problems.

Because of the uncertainty surrounding the effectiveness (for immediate use and long-term prevention) and the toxic repercussions of the employment of these agents, they must be dispensed in an extremely individualized manner to a much greater degree than for common medications such as antibiotics. Consideration must be allowed for personal goals and expectations, type of employment and relationships with supervisors and colleagues, support system, financial status, severity, type and frequency of symptoms, other illnesses, psychological profile, detailed family history, etc. If these are not considered, the benefits of the medications might be marginalized or they may even become dangerous. I have found that few psychiatrists delve into these important factors, perhaps because determining them requires significant time and attention. It should also be expected that modifications to the medication regimen will become necessary over time. This is true not only because some of the aforementioned characteristics change but also due to the introduction of more specific, effective and/or less toxic medications.

Ira: I believe the movement towards the use of medications for the treatment of manic depression has been, on the whole, beneficial. Therefore, I believe Stan has benefited from his pharmacological regimen, but I can't prove it, nor can anyone else, because it is impossible to perform a controlled experiment on Stan or anyone else. However, there are several misconceptions regarding the use and effectiveness of these medications for the treatment of manic depression that results in pernicious consequences for patients, families and the public at large.

The most damaging misconception is that prophylactic medications like lithium work like an antibiotic curing an infection. That is, many believe that the illness can be controlled by simply taking the proper medication. In Chapter 2 I explained that manic depression is highly non-linear. To reiterate, because the physiological mechanisms of manic depression are not understood, it is impossible to accurately predict future developments of the disease for a particular patient. It thus follows that the pharmacological mechanisms associated with the function of any drug are also not understood, making their performance unpredictable. This is true in regard to comparing a drug's performance among several patients and for any individual patient over time. The key point is that it is a grave misconception to assume that the patient is symptom-free just because he is taking medications.

To cite one of many examples during Stan's treatment: after his first manic episode, Stan used lithium for the prophylactic control of his illness. As he described in Chapter 2, he had good days and bad days. But he was able to complete his M.D., Ph.D. and medical internship. It was during his first year of residency that the first of a series of manic episodes would occur, that would eventually end his medical career. It is impossible to know why lithium "worked" and then stopped working for Stan.

This example illustrates another misconception, one held by many psychiatrists. It was often implied to us that Stan went manic because he stopped taking his medication, when, in fact, I know that he went manic before he quit taking his medications. It was the mania itself that made him deny his illness and the effectiveness of the drugs. Put another way, Stan would not stop taking lithium after four-and-a-half years while studying medicine. The fact that he eventually did stop shows that he was not using his normal reasoning, but was manic. This positive feedback loop occurred many more times. The mania would start to affect his thinking, which would cause him to stop taking medication, which would make the mania more intense. To put this issue beyond any question is the fact that when Stan was hospitalized early in a manic episode blood tests revealed that his system still had therapeutic levels of medication.

Another important misconception about the use of medications to control manic depression concerns how they are "tuned." By "tuning" I mean the difficult task of determining what combination of medications, taken at what dosage, at what interval, works best for a particular patient over time. The key difficulty arises from one's inability to read the mind of another, which we discussed in relation to diagnosis. Despite the attempts of the psychiatric profession, as expressed in the *DSM-IV* and many other studies, there is no good method of quantifying behavior. We have found that tuning is a continuous, never-ending process that must be performed with family members who have intimate knowledge of and contact with Stan. I would go so far as to say that it is impossible for a psychiatrist alone to perform this task adequately. Even laboratory tests to determine therapeutic levels of the medication in the blood have proven ineffective in tuning. As implied earlier, the therapeutic levels are more of a measure of toxicity than effectiveness.

A more fundamental understanding of the effectiveness of the long-term prophylactic drugs can be gained by applying the discussion of tuning to questions about their original testing. First of all, how were the data taken? How can therapeutic levels be determined if the output of any experiment is behavior? How is behavior measured? If all the variables that can affect behavior are not known, how can controlled experiments be designed? That is, if no two people have exactly the same environment, or an individual's life is not exactly the same in time, how can there ever be a controlled experiment of a drug's effectiveness? If the illness is nonlinear in time for how long should the studies be conducted? Because there are no good answers to these questions it is impossible to know how well the medications work, which was discussed in a previous question.

A related and problematic issue is determining how any drug treatment can be said to be successful. Stan functioned relatively well on lithium for five years after his first major manic episode before experiencing recurring episodes of mania for several years. Shall we term this lithium treatment a success or a failure? Years later, Stan started prophylactic treatment with valproic acid. He was doing so well that the manufacturer of the drug featured him in its stock report. Three months later he experienced a major episode that resulted in his being fired from his last medical residency position. The point is that a successful treatment can turn into a failure at any time if the reappearance of mania causes the end of a career, financial ruin, the breakup of a marriage or death.

The primary point of my discussion of the pharmacological treatment of manic depression is that it is not a magic bullet. It will be quite problematic until the mechanisms of the illness are understood. Even then I believe treatment will need to include the constant vigilance of loved ones.

Beyond the caveats I have listed above, there is another negative misconception about the use of medications for the treatment of mental diseases. A growing belief, expressed everywhere from serious articles to jokes, is that a significant fraction of the population is being medicated into a state of bliss. The most common culprit for this misconception is the widespread use of Prozac for depression. The belief is that Prozac and other drugs act as narcotics, i.e., mind-altering drugs used for escaping reality. In fact, if used properly, they restore true personality and reality. In this book we have focused on the loss of personality, the appearance of Mr. Hyde, as the fundamental symptom of an unquestionable mental illness in Stan. Associated with the use of medications Stan has been able to regain his personality. On the other hand, the misconceptions described earlier can tend to foster the over-prescription of these medications. This is especially true in the case of treating children, where their baseline personality has not developed, such that it is very uncertain if a genuine, organic mental illness (manic depression in this case) exists at all. The use of medication may well be premature and inappropriate in such cases. Furthermore, there is a host of newly defined behavioral disorders by the psychiatric community which are not considered to be a result of a physical malfunction of the brain. The use of drugs for treatment of these disorders comes too close to medicating away the problems of life instead of helping an individual face them realistically.

chapter five:

the brain and free will

This essay was written in 1990 as an attempt to understand the nature of the brain, behavior, and Stan's illness. Is a person with manic depression ever responsible for his actions? Why do families give up on people with manic depression?

The human brain is a mass called chemical,
Its fate depends on genes and the environmental
In such a state of no free will,
For a piece of candy, a man can kill.

The years 1990-2000 have been designated the Decade of the Brain by the U.S. Congress and signed into law by the president. I suppose this can be considered one of the silly acts that Congress passes every year. But I would rather have them doing silly things than the dreadful things which they do at least as often. In this case I am actually quite interested in their act, for my brother has been living through a nightmarish illness of the brain.

As the galaxy consists of billions of stars and planets, the brain consists of 100 billion neurons, each of which can transmit an electrical or chemical message 80 times a second. The capacity of the neurons to form networks gives the brain a virtually limitless capacity for the storing or processing of information. And like the vast expanse of the cosmos, to a certain extent the brain has been mapped.

It is common knowledge that the left side of the brain processes speech, language comprehension, mathematics and logic while the right side controls nonverbal abilities such as musical and emotional expression, and visual-spatial judgement. The main mass of this "gray matter" is called the cerebrum. However, several other realms of activity have been determined for which specific areas are designated that perform them. Covering the cerebrum is the convoluted tissue of the cortex. The cortex is arranged into columns of cells, different sections of which coordinate voluntary movement, sensation, hearing and speech. The frontal cortex lobe is thought to be critical in creative problem solving. The temporal lobe processes hearing, speech and a sense of personal cognizance. The parietal lobe registers sensory information and communicates with movement-control centers. The occipital lobe processes vision.

Innate aspects of our nature such as emotions, sex and defense drives are held deep within our personalities and governed deep inside the brain by the limbic system. The limbic system is composed of several components. Among the tasks of the hypothalamus are regulation of feeding, fighting and reproduction. The thalmus relays messages from muscles and sense organs. The amygdala serves to process the emotional significance of sensory information. The hippocampus works to convert memory from a temporary to a permanent form.

Beyond the limbic system are the basal ganglia that influence voluntary movement. Finally, there is the cerebellum and the brain stem, located beneath and behind the other structures of the brain. The cerebellum assists in integrating movement while the brain stem is the instinct center that coordinates involuntary activities such as breathing, heart rate and sleep cycles.

As well as the structure and function of the brain much has been learned about disease processes in the brain. In diseases from schizophrenia to dyslexia the malfunctions of particular parts of the brain have been suggested. Diseases as diverse as manic depression and alcoholism are now thought to be caused by particular genetic defects.

This brief, simplistic sketch of the scientific knowledge of the brain makes the point that the brain can be regarded as a chemical machine. It is chemistry that tells your heart to beat, your stomach to eat, or in walking, to move your feet. The drive for sex, the drive for wealth, even simply the drive to drive is the result of some intricate combination of neurotransmitters in action, where the chemistry has been determined by the genetics and environment from which the brain has come forth.

The knowledge of the brain described above is valuable to the medical sciences in determining and treating diseases of the brain. If the chemistry is upset a chemical treatment can fix the disorder. I can attest to the usefulness of this view in the case of my brother. It appears that chemical medications restore his mind. It is the purpose of the Decade of the Brain to promote research in this area.

From a somewhat opposite sense comes the Freudian view that behavior is controlled by the experiences of life. I do not have the knowledge or inclination to describe Freudian psychology adequately but I can say in a simplified exaggeration that it seems to boil down to the premise that your mother's treatment of you at 4 1/2 determines your behavior for the rest of your life.

These two views, say the chemical and the Freudian, dominate the plain of psychological thought. Between them there is a hole, no, a chasm, a Grand Canyon, which separates them while consuming them. For both accept the body while denying the soul.

We have come to the point of this essay. In the Decade of the Brain where is the soul and, more specifically, where is free will? If our behavior is determined by our chemistry or our childhood, is there sin?

I answer yes, there is free will and thus there is sin. The key to the question may be found in the choice of verbs used in the question. I would say behavior is shaped by instead of determined by chemistry and childhood. While these factors influence what we do the final choice is in our hands. Or more precisely, in our souls. The reality is we choose to fast even if our chemistry pushes us to eat. The sins of the flesh are products of choices in the soul. This is the difference between a man and a beast.

I must add that I do believe it is possible to commit sinful acts while in fact not sinning. My brother is a brilliant physician and more importantly a good man who is afflicted with manic depression. While under the control of his mania he does things that he would never do when he is well. It is the evil of this illness that it appropriates his free will. He sins while not sinning. However, I do think he does have some control before he sinks into the mania that can prevent the occurrence of the symptoms. This is where free will comes into play with this disease. For example, some patients choose not to take medication while experiencing depressive lows, even though they understand the negative consequences which may result due to mania. This is especially true for those patients who suffer only from hypomania, where some of the personality and thoughts of the patient remain intact.

People can learn, and must be taught right from wrong, and understand what is lawful behavior. It can be confusing and irritating trying to make a person in a manic state understand these self-evident truths. But it must be understood by those trying to help the patient that it is the illness, not the person, that is noncooperative. It is critical that families understand this, because in the vast majority of cases they must be the primary care givers.

The modern mood is to look for all answers in science even if the questions are not scientific. Just as it has been attempted to take the sin out of crime, we take the mystery out of life. It might seem theoretically possible to explain the chemistry of love. A little hormone here, another one there, and poof, there is love. But what is the tint of blue in the eyes, the curve of a breast, the pitch and volume of a laugh that causes a particular man to love a particular woman? In my opinion this will never be explained by chemistry. This is the mystery of being human.

chapter six:
how does manic depression affect daily life and personal relationships?

---

1. How does manic depression affect daily life?

Stan: Because there is no cure for manic depression it must be monitored and treated for life. Since the onset of symptoms can be extremely rapid and profoundly dangerous, control of the illness must be considered on a daily basis.

To some extent I must think about my disease every day even when I feel perfectly normal. Because of the severity and duration of my manic episodes, when my mind escapes into a different world, I now must question the validity of my interpretation of words and actions closely. This often involves discussing the most ordinary of events with my support system, primarily my family. Fortunately, the basis of reality becomes greater as the time in the stable, non-manic state becomes longer. As much as I may strive to live a pleasant, social and purposeful life, I realize that both my highs and lows can lead to a misreading of the intentions of others and the significance of events. For example, if my mood is abnormally elevated, I have a propensity to discount all my problems. In contrast, when I am in a depressive phase, I tend to take most events too seriously, too personally and from a negative perspective. I must have a special awareness and take precautions about both positive and negative stressful events such as a new job, large purchases, deaths, arguments, etc.

Not only must I make a conscious note of my mood state and the external situation, I must also be aware of and attempt to stabilize basic parameters of human function including sleep, exercise and dietary habits. The amount of sleep I receive has been an indicator of my condition. Functioning at my best I will naturally sleep 9-10 hours comfortably and uninterrupted. While manic I have gone without sleep for days. When I am in a depressed mood, more than anything else, I feel exhausted, sleeping sometimes more than 16 hours per day. This excessive drowsiness is so difficult because its occurrence is unpredictable, impairing my ability to make commitments. Irregular sleep can also indicate the onset of a mood change. I must attempt to go to sleep at the same time each evening as well as wake up at the same hour. If I am sleep-deprived (as in medical residency training) this can induce a high or even full-blown mania. I have also found that sleep deprivation has resulted in depression and the expected excessive tiredness. On days when I feel down and/or more tired, I need to make sure I get up and go at some point to reduce the possibility of a severe depression setting in. When, or if, to force myself to awake isn't always clear to me. Sometimes it is less painful to allow myself to sleep, and the tiredness will abate on its own. At other times I must force myself to arise in order to alleviate more severe symptoms from occurring, including the negative thought processes.

Along the same line, it is extremely important that I get regular exercise or risk symptoms of depression. At times the best I can manage is a walk. Slow thinking, in addition to physical impairment, accompanies my lethargy. I attempt to do light reading, writing or just concentrate on TV to stimulate my thought processes. This brings up an important issue that those with depression hear constantly from others. They see one looking physically healthy, but lethargic, and thus lazy. A typical remark I have heard is to "snap out of it." The person who uses this kind of motivation does not understand the nature of the illness. Unfortunately, there is no simple answer for the loved one as to when or if to push the mildly depressed patient and if so to what extent. The support system must recognize that the patient's inability to perform tasks is part of the disease.

My diet is another indicator of mood changes that I must carefully monitor and manage. I have maintained a well-regulated, low-calorie and low-fat diet for most of my adult life. This has been prompted by my medical training in cardiology and the predisposition to heart disease in our family. During mood changes, especially associated with depression, I have lost control of my eating habits to such an extent that I once, in the process of recovering from a manic episode, experienced a weight gain that was 50% of my reduced total body weight (from 100 to 150 lbs.) in one month.

I have attempted to track my mood and sleep on a daily basis through a quantitative measure (for example, assigning 1 for a very depressed state and 10 for being manic) in order to minimize or forestall adverse behavior. Unfortunately, I have found this technique to be of little value. The onset of mania can develop so quickly that tracking did not give me adequate warning. While depressed, I found even this small task to be too arduous. Having a member of the support system chart this information would probably be more effective because of greater objectivity. The recording of these data may show a pattern of change that may be cyclical or the result of certain external stimuli, and this could be of help in treatment. Of course, the psychiatrist should seek this information, be it quantitative or qualitative, from both the patient and support members.

In conclusion, the cause and effects of the illness are often difficult to discern. For example did a decrease in sleep cause the manic symptoms or was the decrease in sleep a result of the mania? Whatever the case may be, it is always prudent to monitor the above parameters of daily function and try to maintain their normalcy.

Ira: If you have read this book through to this point you understand that manic depression is an all-encompassing disease which may affect every aspect of life on a daily basis. The impact on personal life is critical because it is the relationships with family and friends that must be maintained, if not strengthened, since they form the support group that must be in place to treat the disease. Consequently, the personal life of the family is also fundamentally affected, more than is the case with other major illnesses. The questions and answers in this chapter will illustrate how the disease is manifested in the personal and daily lives of patients and their families.

2. Do you always take medication?

Stan: To emphatically reiterate, manic depression is a lifelong illness without a cure. Current available medications have been "proven effective" by physicians who claim expertise in treating this disorder. I and almost all psychiatrists and patients consider these agents as vital to treating this disease, which is considered one of the most amenable to medication of all the psychiatric illnesses. Therefore, I take medication every day and realize this will be required for the remainder of my life (unless there is some therapeutic breakthrough). I now articulate one of the most important messages in this book: having a support system is always necessary, usually far more important than the drug therapy in controlling this illness. Despite taking medication, I realize there is a possibility that these medications have no effect on the course of the illness. This is because of the inherent nature of the difficulty in scientifically evaluating this behavioral disease. This can be especially disconcerting considering the substantial cost of many of these drugs. The medication(s) and doses are based on the perceived benefit of preventing the symptoms as opposed to the adverse side effects of the medications. The tuning of the medications is far from an exact science, as we discussed in Chapter 4.

When stable I have always diligently taken my medication, rarely missing even a single dose. However, on almost every occasion when there has been a relapse (because of the inability of the medication to prevent the recurrence of symptoms), I have subsequently stopped taking medications. This is because, in the manic state, I falsely believed that I was in perfect health and that these drugs were ineffectual (being nothing but placebo or sugar pills). It is interesting to note that my psychiatrists have attributed the mania to a conscious decision on my part to discontinue the medication. Thus, they falsely believe the medication is always effective and inappropriately blame me, the patient, for the relapse.

Ira: The fact that Stan must take medication on a daily basis for the rest of his life is assumed to be a terrible burden by everyone to whom I have spoken about his care. However, as I tell Stan, there are many tasks that are not particularly enjoyable but which we must perform every day. Most of us go to the bathroom, brush our teeth and take vitamins every day. Is taking medication for manic depression that much greater a burden? Perhaps, but in this instance I believe looking at this situation in the best light possible is appropriate. However, there is an aspect of taking any medication that was not adequately appreciated by any of the physicians who have treated Stan. They have taken the euphemism of calling the negative effects caused by medications as "side" effects to heart. The reality that the negative effects can have a "primary" impact on health and quality of life was ignored by the psychiatrists.

3. How does manic depression affect work relationships?

Stan: When in a manic state I am incapable of functioning in society, let alone in the workplace. If I am suffering from depressions, the tiredness and slow thinking also make work extremely difficult, if not impossible.

However, if I am in good control and have a professional position which can allow for days in which I need more rest because of either stress or tiredness, I believe I can be productive. The proof of that assessment is this book. A supportive environment is necessary for success in most job-related situations. In practice, this means that coworkers must also be friends. Some professions might require less support from colleagues because the demands of the work are less taxing and time requirements are more flexible.

Manic depression affects the educated professional as well as those in other jobs. Because professionals generally have higher incomes and more responsibility and have established a greater reputation in the community, the ramifications of the illness can be more damaging. It is difficult to regain the previous societal standing following symptoms of depression and especially mania. Greater education may also be manifested in the mania itself. For example, my writing capability coupled with my knowledge resulted in my composing sociopolitical tracts much like the Unabomber.

It is not easy to find support on the job unless a friendship proceeded employment. I thought that when I entered a psychiatry residency program I would finally be given support in the workplace because they certainly understood this illness. In stark contrast to my expectations, this group deliberately made my experience more taxing than that of my peers before firing me. This discrimination toward me and my illness was made even more obvious by comparing it to the treatment of another resident who had a heart ailment. Despite missing many days, this individual with a physical ailment was offered nothing but compassion and leniency by the department faculty.

Ira: I have discussed Stan's illness with every employer he has had since his first major manic episode. From these discussions, and through assessing the actions of these employers, I have come to the conclusion that the prospects for understanding and support from them are very slim. This is actually very understandable. If loved ones find it overwhelmingly difficult and frustrating to cope with the illness, why should we expect it to be any different for acquaintances made through work? For Stan, only the friendships he made before the onset of the illness as a student at the Medical University of South Carolina at Charleston were able to withstand the devastation of his manic behavior. These friends helped him receive care when he was manic and gave him moral support when he recovered. In every other case, little or no attempt was made to help him, and he was eventually fired. Were these actions due to ignorance of the disease? No, Stan was always employed in some aspect of medicine. Even a thorough understanding of manic depression in particular has not made a difference. At the onset of a manic episode Stan was summarily fired from a psychiatry residency position. In other words, he was fired for being ill with a disease that his supervisors treated every day. This being the case, in what everyday occupations should a person with manic depression expect any understanding of this misunderstood illness? Is this fair? Of course not, but it is understandable. We cannot, nor should we, expect people to be so altruistic as to act like saints. I do not suggest laws be passed against this unfairness because public policy that runs against the fundamental facts of human nature is bound to fail.

4. Are there any positive symptoms of manic depression such as increased productivity or artistic creativity?

Stan: This question was stimulated by the common belief that people with this disease produce more when in the hypomanic state and by the work of author, psychologist, researcher and patient Kay Redfield Jamison. Dr. Jamison suggests that the very definition of hypomania demonstrates the advantageous qualities of rapidity and clarity of thought, decisiveness and increased energy.

I would like to comment on two stages of my mania. The first is one in which I am revved up but my judgment is sound. I suppose it is similar to a state some try to achieve by drinking coffee or taking caffeine pills. I frequently observed this in others as they prepare for a test or have a morning jolt of coffee to start the day. I find this state of mind and energy to be uncomfortable. I'm less deliberate and more prone to make mistakes, though it is possible that there is some increase in my rate of accomplishment. This is especially true with respect to my depressions, which often preceded and would then follow this state.

The second stage (which the question directly refers to) that I have suffered from is episodes of hypomania. These periods of increased energy were on occasion noted by others in contact with me and associated with a decline in judgment. They were rare and most often escalated into mania. The energy from this state actually decreased constructive productivity. I might accomplish more, but the quality would be poor based on false premises resulting from my impaired judgment. For instance, I might read a large number of medical publications in a short time span, but the conclusions I would draw would be inaccurate at minimum and possibly ludicrous.

Some may look at this disease as almost a good thing, given the number of prominent poets, painters and composers who seemingly have benefited from manic depression. However, I believe that artistic creativity is, overall, decreased if not significantly hampered as a consequence of this disease. To be sure, during mania, you certainly view the world differently from others and your usual self, but the vast majority of these thoughts are ridiculous. On the other hand, there is the potential to see the world differently than others in a normal state of mind. In addition, experiences are expanded on account of this mindset. For example, I traveled to other cities, dealt with police, ate differently, etc. I also have noted an enhancement or alteration in the sensual functions of taste and hearing. It is possible that a small number of these manic memories could be harnessed in some creative way.

Ira: The work of Kay Jamison on this subject is very intriguing and in many ways quite persuasive. However, I have reservations about the conclusion that manic depression is a source of artistic creativity. My first concern might be categorized as aesthetic. Certainly it is true that the manic state allows one to produce great amounts of material. In the manic state one also perceives the world from different perspectives, which could provide insight into artistic creation. But to me art can only be good in proportion to its reflection of the reality of the human condition. This is even true for such abstract art as music. A fundamental mark of mania is the loss of reality for the individual. I would say that the great artists who suffered from manic depression, such as Van Gogh, were not great because of the illness, but in spite of the illness. A second reservation concerns the conclusion that manic depression can have a positive consequence. To put it succinctly, a malfunctioning, sick organ cannot benefit the patient. I believe the increase in productivity sometimes associated with manic depression, perhaps during hypomania, is misunderstood. Certainly during a depression it is terribly difficult to accomplish anything, and so when the depression ends it seems that the manic period results in productivity. But I think it is just the absence of depression that is the key to being healthy and productive.

I also question the interpretation of Jamison's data. In a scholarly analysis, she shows that there is a much higher percentage of creative people who suffer from manic depression than of those in the more mundane professions.   An obvious conclusion is that manic depression aids creativity.   But there can be another interpretation.   Suppose a brilliant young artist and a brilliant young banker each experiences their first manic episode at the age of 25. They both are committed to a mental hospital and require six months to recover. I think most would agree that the banker's career would be crippled. Certainly the artist's career would also be curtailed, but he does not have the day-to-day responsibilities of the average profession. Thus, there is a filtering effect of patients with manic depression in most professions. In fact, the artistic professions are among the few professions where extended absences are not devastating to future prospects.

5. How is the family affected by manic depression?

Ira: I believe Stan would now be living on the street, in a hospital, in jail or even be dead if he did not have the support and care of his family. Because of this belief I also think that the participation of the family is crucial in the treatment and care of manic depression. To perform this role, the family members must understand the nature of this illness and be aware of their own feelings regarding their sick loved ones. Unfortunately, many families find this task too onerous to perform.

Why do families give up on their loved ones? The term in vogue to explain this phenomenon is "burden." Many people have commented that Stan's illness must be such a burden to me. In support-group meetings I often heard the frustration expressed by parents, siblings and spouses about their sick children, brothers, sisters, husbands and wives. In particular, they felt their efforts at assistance were unappreciated and ineffective. This response reflects the fundamental, insidious nature of this disease, as manifested in the character of Mr. Hyde. In thinking about how to understand the behavior of Stan and other people who suffer from mental illness I wrote the essay on the brain and free will which is Chapter 5.

As an example of how a family's misunderstanding of mental illness can have tragic consequences, consider the story of the Franklin family reported in the September 4, 2000 issue of *Time* magazine. Shaka, the young son of Les Franklin, committed suicide in 1990 at the age of 16. Mr. Franklin, a successful corporate executive, channeled his grief into the founding of the Shaka Franklin Foundation for Youth, which is dedicated to the prevention of youth suicide. In 2000, Shaka's older brother Jamon committed suicide. Les' reaction to this tragedy was not so positive, as described in the *Time* article:

"Jamon's death, however, has made Franklin furious. 'I know he never got over his brother's death, his baby brother, six years apart,' Les told *Time* shortly after discovering Jamon's body. 'But he promised me that he'd never hurt me the way his brother hurt me, and in the final analysis he broke his promise, and I'm very angry.' He adds, 'There will be no Jamon's place. Shaka was 16; he was a baby. Jamon was a 31-year-old man. I'm not going to give him that. He knew I loved him. He made a horrible, horrible decision.'"

Unfortunately, it is obvious that Mr. Franklin does not understand the nature of the mental illness that took the lives of his sons. The fact that two people in the same family committed suicide points to genetically based clinical depression. It was reported that Jamon battled with bouts of depression and irregular sleep. The point of bringing up this painful anecdote is that even someone immersed in understanding mental illness like Mr. Franklin does not understand the illnesses of his own sons. Thus the familiar tragedy due to mental illness is repeated: the victim is ultimately blamed for his actions.

My attitude has always been based on stoicism and the knowledge that however burdensome my responsibilities to my family might be, they have only been a fraction of the burden that Stan has had to endure dealing with the illness himself. My message to the family is that there is a serious job to be done, and you are the only ones capable of performing it.

The greatest effect on the family is the loss of the basic personality of their loved one to Mr. Hyde. Since the onset of Stan's illness our mother has always related to any celebrity, such as Bill Cosby, whose child had died. By understanding that Mr. Hyde was not Stan, the brother whom I loved and wanted to help, I did not have the sense of being unappreciated.

In a more fundamental manner, taking care of my responsibilities as Stan's brother has been an innate response to family life. What does it mean to do good in life if not carrying the appropriate "burdens"? A friend of mine recommended I read Wally Lamb's novel *I Know This Much is True*. The novel follows the mental state of a man whose twin brother is schizophrenic. For most of the book the healthy brother cannot deal with the pain, anger, guilt and

assorted other emotions he feels due to the illness of his brother. Eventually he does gain the
wisdom, through the aid of a psychologist, that
it is much better to face life's trials with courage
and virtue than self-pity and vice. But this has
been known for centuries in all cultures, except
perhaps our own. For example, it is expressed
by the great Indian writer Nirad Chaudhuri, in
this passage from the second volume of his
autobiography, *Thy Hand, Great Anarch! India
1921-1952:*

"I have learnt the significance of suffering
without understanding why it should be the lot
of human beings to have it inflicted on them. It
does not regard innocence, nor wrongdoing, but
comes upon all impartially. It seems to be some
natural, inescapable phenomenon like storms,
floods, earthquakes, or volcanic eruptions.
Looking upon it in this light, I have come to feel
that there is nothing more cowardly than to
nurse a grievance for it. Above all, I have come
to hold that it is frivolity of the worst kind to air
cheap compassion over it. There are only two
victories over suffering offered to man: either to
rise above it or to submit to it without complaining. That is being *Homo sapiens* in the first
instance."

On the other hand, I certainly understand
how people can feel overwhelmed by this ill-

ness. First of all, manic depression is so difficult to understand. The fundamental purpose of
this book is to enhance understanding. Dealing
with manic depression is also very time-con-
suming for the family members who must be
able to live their own lives in a healthy way. This
can more readily be accomplished if the whole
family takes up part of the responsibility. And
finally, of supreme importance, it must be
understood that second-guessing actions taken
in good faith, including the inevitable failures, is
nonproductive. Sometimes nothing can even be
attempted. Many times all approaches are
bound to fail, but you can never know for sure.
Personally I do not feel guilty or morose in these
instances, because I understand that I cannot
help Stan if my own life is unhealthy.

6. What must the family do?

Ira: There are three fundamental stages of
the illness that require different kinds of attention from the family: psychotic manic episodes,
periods of recovery from mania including
depression, and healthy periods.

The onset of a psychotic manic episode was
like a hurricane blowing through our family.
Even if it did not cause great damage it certain-

ly disrupted life. Of course we have described how devastating these episodes were for Stan. Our mother's mental health was also damaged by a combination of depression and panic disorder that was set off by Stan's danger. Her agitation disrupted my attempts to handle these difficult situations. Therefore, I usually tried to shield from her the specifics of Stan's condition and what I was doing to help him, while simultaneously comforting her. The overall goal of my efforts was to get Stan into a safe environment where treatment could be initiated. This was usually the hospital. An account given in Chapter 1 of one such episode, when Stan traveled to Hawaii, was typical of my efforts to help him and my mother's condition. This essay relates my experiences dealing with the personal and societal hurdles that must be overcome to assist a mentally ill individual.

After a manic episode Stan was left weakened mentally, physically, emotionally, financially and just about every other way. Furthermore, he was overwhelmed by side effects to the antipsychotic medications, such as Haldol, initiated in an effort to bring him out of the mania. He needed to be supported in all of these areas as we nursed him back to strength. Following discharge from the hospital he would live with a member of the family so we could take care of all of his essential needs. Perhaps the most difficult aspect of this recovery was living through the akathisia due to Haldol, or other antipsychotic medications. Akathisia is persistent restlessness which may sound benign but was like torture to Stan. We would take walks, go on drives and see movies, anything that might reduce that terrible feeling. He would also require assistance with financial, legal and career difficulties that I would attempt to resolve. A discussion of these difficulties is provided in Chapter 8. The normal melancholia of dealing with the humiliation and loss associated with each episode was sometimes accompanied by bouts of clinical depression in the form of crying spells. Medications were used to alleviate these symptoms, but I think more important was our role giving Stan moral support in a manner such that he would never doubt that we would always be there for him.

Manic depression is manifested in abnormal behavior. The critical task the family should perform during healthy periods is the assessment of behavior on a regular if not daily basis. In effect they should act as thought police to catch Mr. Hyde before he does any damage. Make no mistake, this prophylactic assistance is an extremely difficult and onerous task. Being a thought policeman is difficult because it requires many years of observation of the particular individual to be able to discern the onset of mania. It is onerous because it requires the restricting of the freedom of a person who normally is perfectly reasonable. Especially in our liberated society it is problematical to question the motives of anyone. Personally, I always wanted to be optimistic, and so Stan's hypomania deteriorated into psychotic mania on several occasions due to my inaction.

The methods used to determine abnormal thoughts and the course of corrective action must be tailored to each individual and perhaps will change for an individual over time. I will describe the methods that we have come to understand are useful for Stan. When Stan is manic he has certain mannerisms which are not part of his normal demeanor. He tends to furrow his brow, stare intently, cross his legs and ask questions like a demented David Frost. He will do this especially in response to a question posed to him about his own health. Perhaps nothing is more indicative of the onset of mania as when he begins to deny the existence of his illness. He may simply pause before answering a question regarding his health. Or he might attribute his abnormal behavior to another cause besides manic depression. For example, while we were writing this book, Stan experienced a minor manic episode. He added this paragraph after my answer to Chapter 2, question 2, where I described how I erroneously had attributed his abnormal behavior to the stress of medical school.

Stan: I believe you were correct to incriminate medical school in my behavior pattern. Although I am pleased to have completed this rigorous curriculum, it is arduous despite what anyone may say to the contrary. I know of no one who has ever gone through this process unscathed. The manifestations might be increased smoking, lack of exercise, poor diet, impotence, irritability and/or high blood pressure, culminating eventually in serious, possibly life-threatening results. The point is that the situation is a cauldron that will explode in one manner or another.

Ira: Notice that Stan is giving reasons for his behavior other than the illness, and implying that it is typical for everyone to experience similar problems. The upshot is that the disease manic depression is not the cause. And yet he wrote this paragraph for a book about manic depression!

As the Hawaii chapter shows, it is apparent that during a psychotic manic episode, beyond Stan's immediate safety, another focus of my efforts was to maintain his financial well-being and career opportunities. This was also true during his healthy periods. I never wanted him to feel I was checking up on him. Furthermore, I wanted to help him in a way such that he would not be denied his independence and normality. For example, I always helped Stan move to a new city to restart his career. I usually did not directly question him about his health. In a way, the normal mode of our relationship was denial, because it was a painful subject for both of us. For more than ten years I had literally chased Stan around the country to contain his manic episodes. In the end, the attempt to maintain Stan's independence and normality failed because he experienced repeated manic episodes that shattered his career and finances. Thus, a key question must be faced: how independent can a manic depressive patient be? From the complete independence of a healthy person, to the severe restrictions of life in a mental hospital, there is a continuous range of possibilities in response to this question.

Eventually to gain greater control of his care, I suggested that Stan move to San Antonio, where I lived, instead of pursuing the best position possible. I had also obtained power of attorney over Stan's assets to be able to take over his affairs in the event of another episode. He began a psychiatry residency at the University of Texas Health Science Center at San Antonio several months after joining me there.

Unfortunately, this increased level of control was not sufficient to prevent another major psychotic episode from occurring. Stan was fired from his position and was in denial of his illness. At this point I decided to take a different, but more dangerous approach than I had taken for the previous ten years. I did not make any effort to have Stan committed, but allowed the mania to dissipate his resources sufficiently so that society would intervene to force treatment. This was dangerous for all of the reasons we have previously described. But I believed that allowing Stan to flounder in his independence would now help me apply restrictions as necessary in the future. Furthermore, his career and finances had already been damaged to such an extent that, at least temporarily, I abandoned efforts to help him in these areas to concentrate on maintaining his health.

I had expected that Stan would be picked up by the police within six months because of his odd behavior or his lack of money to pay for the things he still wanted. I think that there is truth in the adage that society treats someone behaving oddly with money as an eccentric and someone poor as crazy. Sadly, the police only placed Stan in a hospital more than two years after his psychotic episode began. Our interactions with the police and the rest of society during this period of Stan's psychotic state are discussed in Chapter 8.

Since Stan's recovery we have instituted a new regime of restrictions to protect him from the damage of another manic episode. His financial freedom is severely restricted, to the point that he has no money or assets of his own. He has put his career on hold for the time being to concentrate on maintaining his health. Perhaps most important, Stan has regular discussions about his health with me.

The success of this new approach of restricted freedom was demonstrated when Stan experienced a minor manic episode that was not allowed to spiral out of control. I was able to recognize his manic thoughts in this case through the work he was doing on this book, as shown by Stan's passage in the previous question. We were able to discuss the change in his condition, increase his dose of antipsychotic medication and suspend his work on the book. This mild manic episode was thus short-lived and benign. I must add, however, that even at that time, with all of our experience, it was still difficult talking to Stan about his mania when he was manic. It also took several months to begin writing again, because it appeared that working on this book aggravated his condition, or was even the cause of the relapse.

In summary, the family must provide support in virtually all aspects of life and must also institute a regime of restrictions for the patient's safety. I believe these restrictions are analogous to restricting the freedom of children to play on a busy street; it is instigated for their own safety. But it is difficult to achieve the optimal level of restrictions. Most of my efforts to help Stan eventually failed. Yet I don't think it was wrong to try and give Stan as much freedom to live his life normally for as long as possible. Even the approach we are using today may need to be altered in the future.

7. How does manic depression affect personal relationships?

Stan: This is a very important topic. Hopefully, when stable and under the best of circumstances, it has little to no effect. But the sometimes subtle and not-so-subtle symptoms directly affect relationships. In my experience, this was more evident prior to my diagnosis of manic depression. Poor judgment and the loss of one's usual personality can have severe adverse consequences. I made statements similar to what a drunk might say that harmed my relationships with others. This tapered off for me once the diagnosis was established because I became much more careful and deliberate in my interactions with others. With time and continued stability, I have learned to essentially speak for myself, not Mr. Hyde. The exception is that I must be very careful when I feel tense or uneasy about a conversation. These instances require that I consult with my support system for the validity of my thinking.

One of the most difficult effects of this disease on relationships is trying to make people understand that some of my limitations (for example, being unable to arise for an early appointment) and circumstances in life (being unemployed) are due to this disease. Unfortunately, this illness is extremely difficult to comprehend even if one is familiar with it. Thus it takes a great deal of time to explain. Even after a long discussion(s) only a small percentage of people will grasp its full implications. Because it is a psychiatric disorder, it also carries a strong negative connotation of craziness to most people because mental illness is still pervasively misunderstood. Furthermore, as with any illness, patients also want to maintain some confidentiality about their medical history. Why should an acquaintance know if you have a history of a bleeding ulcer, for instance? The constellation of all these factors makes it difficult to determine to whom to divulge, to what extent and when in the relationship to discuss the matter. There are no absolutes. I have learned that it is pivotal to establish yourself as a genuine human being with a normal personality first. If not, the patient faces the potential consequence of being looked at only as the person with the disease, which interferes with developing a positive reputation and relationships.

Even if I believe I have developed a strong friendship with someone and he or she has the capacity to understand this psychiatric illness in an educated and non-judgmental manner, I still have reservations about discussing my illness. This is because the information then becomes more likely to be spread to others who don't understand as well. Although I know who I am and am proud of my character, my reputation is still important to me. I want to be treated at with respect yet, I realize that others will consider me in a different manner if they become aware I have a mental illness. I must restate that the vast majority of the public thinks that if you have a psychiatric illness you are of deficient character. For example, if I tell people that I went on spending sprees as a consequence of my illness, they rarely can comprehend that my loss of self-control was not due to a character flaw. I recognize that in publishing this book I am divulging to the public my illness and its consequences to my life, but this is with the hope that I may help many others. Furthermore, understanding, through the full explanation of the illness documented here, may reduce the possibility of negative prejudices to myself.

Relationships with the opposite sex are especially sensitive because of the illness. Whenever there is an emotionally charged situation of either a positive or negative nature, a heightened awareness of symptoms must ensue. A close or intimate relationship invariably produces such feelings. Having the illness and the associated roller coaster of symptoms has made it extremely difficult for me to sustain such a relationship. Other environmental circumstances in my life have also contributed to this difficulty. These include the long educational period requiring significant attention and time, as well as delayed financial independence. I have found it difficult to determine when to tell someone I had been dating that I suffer from this illness. When I was first diagnosed, my psychiatrist told me to reveal it on the second date. This advice seems arbitrary because it might prematurely end a potentially excellent match. Indeed, this has happened to me. Therefore, I use the same discretion I discussed above regarding divulging this personal medical history to friends. However, there is no question that if the relationship becomes serious, my partner will be told about this important aspect of my life.

On a social level, for the most part, my friends remained friends when I was first diagnosed. However, they did not understand what I coped with because of this disease. Therefore, I receive little support from them. Perhaps this book will strengthen some of my friendships. Because I was still in the training portion of my career and not settled, I was not in close contact for a prolonged period with anyone. Then I suffered from severe bouts of mania that destroyed much of my life. This included separation from my friends. Even though I am now stable, my current unemployed status makes it uncomfortable for me to contact my old friends from college and medical school.

I am sorry to report that I have received no support whatsoever from my former colleagues in the medical profession outside of those who knew me before my diagnosis. I have seen many instances where they offer significant help to those with physical illnesses. But mental illness does not summon such attention. In the psychiatry program I entered, I specifically made them aware of my condition so that I would receive support; yet, as I described earlier, no attempt was made to help me. This is no doubt in part because these colleagues were not my friends first, who knew me as a competent colleague, not as an illness. They mistook my behavior in the diseased state as part of my personality and/or my illness was too much of a burden. In contrast, a physical heart ailment in another resident was not.

As I have witnessed with respect to my family, it is easier for them to talk to others about the illness in me than it is for myself. However the family is not directly under judgment. It is true that some families do not wish to discuss the subject because it may tarnish them. Some families, for instance, will not reveal the occurrence of a suicide. In the very writing of this work, I find it more difficult to discuss this illness and my experiences than it is for Ira. There are two reasons for this. First, the memories that are rekindled can be painful. Second, I have some reservations about revealing some of these personal tragedies. Nevertheless, I do write this because I believe my experiences are not unique. By discussing them, I address what I have found to be the best way to lead a fulfilling life, despite previous problems and the continued presence of the disease.

The topic of my illness usually comes up when I am asked what I do for a living. In our culture this is a defining aspect of a person and is almost always asked when one is first introduced to someone. Since numerous individuals with this illness are on disability, as I currently am, it can be difficult to avoid mentioning the disease. However, as I said earlier, this is confidential. Some older people with the disease respond by stating that they are retired. Because I hope my unemployment is temporary, my psychiatrist suggested that I say I am on sabbatical. However, many people outside of the academic world don't know what a sabbatical is. Thus, I usually respond by explaining that I am a physician. If more questions arise, I mention my specialty as neurology. If there is further inquiry about where my practice is located, I respond that I am working on a research project (this book). A few people ask about the topic of this work and I respond that I am pursuing a neurobiological or neuropsychiatric investigation. Occasionally the question becomes even more specific and I will mention that the topic is manic depression.

Ira: The major effect of Stan's illness on our family has been to bring it closer together. This is true literally in that we have spent much, much more time together than we otherwise would have. It is also true in that we have had much deeper conversations about many other things that are important to us. However, if we were not all committed to help Stan, I think the illness would have torn our family apart. The fact that neither our other brother, Mike, nor I had our own families allowed us to more easily meet our responsibilities to Stan. Thus, Stan's illness did not have a major impact on my other relationships. However, in many ways this book is the inspiration and fruit of my many discussions with my friends and other acquaintances about my experiences helping Stan cope with his illness. It is something I could not hide because in so many cases an emergency would force me to alter the plans I had made for attending a ball game, going on a trip or simply going out for a drink. Through my discussions it became clear that dealing with mental health problems is relatively common and that the insights I have gained through my experience could be valuable to others.

chapter seven:
how bureaucracy fails those with
manic depression?

When Bob Dole lost the 1996 presidential election he returned home to Russell, KS to a parade in his honor. Well, at least he did so in a television commercial. Of course everybody knew him, even the clerk who was handling his purchase. But she still required him to present his identification before she would cash his check. The commercial was amusing because everyone has been in a similar situation where the rule comes before thought, before even the obvious. Unfortunately, the characteristics of mental illness, especially manic depression, force patients and loved ones to interact with many bureaucracies, both public and private, where this "clerk mentality" is prevalent. These interactions can be extremely frustrating because manic depression is a human problem that requires judgment by those with intimate knowledge of the patient in its treatment. Bureaucracies are specifically designed to function with minimal judgment; therefore, they provide inadequate care or even exacerbate problems. This essay will discuss this fundamental inconsistency based on my experiences helping my brother deal with manic depression. My personal frustration with bureaucracies was greatly diminished once I understood their character. Furthermore, this knowledge enabled me to direct situations toward the care I knew was in his best interest. But in fact, it was even in the best interest of those members of the bureaucracy. It is my hope that this essay may guide readers in the same fashion.

First consider the nature of a bureaucracy. As organizations become large (though everything discussed here might also apply to a group as small as two people) a method of management must be put in place to direct individuals in the organization towards its goals. A minimal management approach would simply state the goal with no direction as to how the goal should be achieved. But typically there are many rules employed to constrain individual behavior. As the number of constraints increases, the role of individual judgment decreases. In effect, individuals are taught not to think.

The "clerk mentality" is widespread and for good reason. The advantage to the clerk for thinking is minimal to nonexistent when his thought results in a positive consequence. This is true because those positive consequences are usually difficult to measure in that they may be no more than what a customer or client expects. Bob Dole would not have noticed if the clerk simply accepted his check. However, penalties for wrong decisions, especially when they break a rule, are severe. So when you ask a clerk to break a rule, even in an obvious situation where the rule does not apply, realize that for the clerk there is the potential for only pain and no gain.

In a similar fashion to the development of rules to direct performance, standards must be implemented to judge performance. By and large these standards attempt to be objective by using quantifiable measures of performance. For example, for a sales clerk in a store the counting measure might be the number of sales. Not included in this measure of performance is how fellow workers are treated or if dishonesty and pressure are used to increase sales. Even when subjective measures of quality are considered almost always the quantifiable measure becomes the dominant one. In a profession as distinguished as academia, it is the number of papers published that has become the dominant measure of scholarship, not necessarily the quality of them.

This atmosphere where thought and initiative are punished and where counting statistics are the only measures of performance results in bored workers who avoid all effort other than that directed towards improving the "count." Here is the source of frustration in the typical interaction with a bureaucracy.

On the other hand, is there any other way to run a large organization like a corporation or the government? Usually the rules are very sensible. Many people pass fraudulent checks, therefore merchants require identification. Make it a rule because, to be honest, some clerks have poor judgment about these things. And anyway, shouldn't everyone be carrying identification? Certainly we take pride in our justice system when it follows the rule of law, that is, rules that apply all the time and to everyone regardless of his station in life.

So we live in a society where large organizations provide many useful functions but must create bureaucracies to run them. In most cases this arrangement is reasonable and beneficial, even with the aggravations and drawbacks described above. However, there are some problems where bureaucracies are inevitably ineffective or even counterproductive. These are the problems related to the unique nature of individuals. I call them "human problems." Three important human problems in any society are raising children, helping the poor and treating mental illness.

Imagine creating a set of rules for the raising of children. Should children be guided for a profession from a young age, like Tiger Woods, or allowed to find their own way? Should a child be punished for an F grade or given encouragement? The answer to these questions is, as all parents know, "it depends." It depends on more factors about the individual child than I can list in this short essay which parents take into account in the multitude of day-to-day decisions associated with raising children. Raising children is one of the fundamental human problems (perhaps "joys" is a more appropriate noun than "problems") in society.

A man and his family live in a town that is devastated by a flood. He has lost his house and his job. A different young man, the graduate of a fine college, quits his job after receiving a sizable inheritance. After a couple of years he has frittered away all of his money on pleasure such that he is bankrupt. Should both of these poor people receive cash assistance? Perhaps this is an extreme example but makes the point that the poor are individuals with unique stories and needs. The historian Gertrude Himmelfarb has described the Victorian sentiment that there are deserving and undeserving poor. The Victorians were correct, and they had much success helping the poor, as Himmelfarb has documented. It requires judgment to help the poor such that they can succeed in life and not simply take advantage of a handout or become dependent on a welfare check.

Now let us examine the human problem that is the focus of this essay, treating mental illness, in particular manic depression. Manic depression is an extremely difficult illness to manage because it is what I call nonlinear. The patient goes through periods of depression and euphoria that often become psychotic. The effects of this illness are felt in virtually every aspect of a person's life, including the personal, social, financial, legal and professional, as well as the medical. It is very difficult to predict how particular patients will react to a particular treatment or to their particular environment at any particular time. Thus, any particular rule designed for the general public is usually detrimental to containing the consequences of the illness. Even rules specifically designed to deal with the mentally ill are usually ineffective or counterproductive. Thus, bureaucracies are not up to the task of considering the implications of manic depression, because this dehumanizing disease is to the greatest extent a human problem.

A key difficulty lies in the atmosphere of the legal system, which through decades of jurisprudence is favorable towards recognizing only the rights of the atomized individual. Mediating institutions, of which by far the most important is the family, are most often put off in their attempts to influence care. This is a critical shortcoming of the system because it is vital to have an understanding of the patient's normal personality and history to facilitate treatment. Furthermore, it is only the family that can provide the long-term care and support necessary to achieve a productive life. No paid employee will ever have the fortitude or opportunity to properly assist a patient with manic depression. It can be said that the patience of love is necessary in the long term assistance of the mentally ill.

I have experienced many examples of the clerk mentality in attempting to help my brother cope with manic depression, which were excused by claiming civil rights for the patient.

This was especially true when attempting to detain him for treatment. While in a manic, psychotic state the safest place for my brother, the place where treatment could begin, was the mental hospital. But getting him committed was always difficult, many times because I did not know where to find him. In those cases I would attempt to track him down through his credit- or debit-card purchases. Even with a power of attorney I had obtained for just this kind of situation it was only a 50-50 chance that I would be given any information. You see, this was a very unusual request that required a decision on the part of the employees that went against the rules of divulging private information. This is the kind of decision that a "good" clerk will always try to avoid. But it depends upon the individual; some clerks still think.

You might think the police would be helpful in locating a sick mental-health patient. On the contrary, the police are imbued with the clerk mentality. They invariably find a reason not to do anything. Helping get mentally ill people to the hospital is not one of the counting statistics used to grade their performance. In their bureaucracy only when the patient is deemed "dangerous to himself or others" will the police assist in hospitalization. In general they have a minimal understanding of mental illness and would prefer to not get involved. If they weren't a part of a bureaucracy, but were members of the community and knew the patient and family, assistance would be readily available.

After my brother was located, the problem was getting him into the hospital and keeping him there. On some occasions he would go with me voluntarily, but during other manic episodes he was uncooperative, so I would attempt to have him committed to the hospital involuntarily. Everyone who in any way must deal with the mentally ill knows that the criteria for commitment are being "dangerous to himself or others." But my brother was never violent, so I had great difficulty getting him committed to the hospital. Because of my understanding of the workings of the judicial bureaucracy in his most recent episode, my strategy was to observe the situation as best I could while waiting for him to run out of money. Then it would be society that would deem him dangerous, for a person is considered dangerous if he does not pay his bills. I was in contact with the management at his apartment so I knew that he had stopped paying his rent. I was in favor of evicting him to force a confrontation with the police, the end result being his admittance to the hospital. But unfortunately this involuntary hospitalization did not occur because he abandoned his apartment and left town due to manic thoughts. Thus, there would be no confrontation with the police when the eviction took place. In a standard eviction the furniture is simply moved on to the curb. It was obvious that his possessions needed to be tended to rather than discarded. While the apartment manager was cooperative, the lawyer who represented the complex demonstrated the clerk mentality. I offered to continue paying the rent or to have the furniture moved at a later date. But this did not fit the usual practice, so it was not considered by the lawyer. Annoyed by my persistence in trying to save my brother's possessions, he asked me, "Are you your brother's keeper?" This biblical reference could not have been more ironic, for indeed, God created us to be our brothers' keepers.

My brother left his apartment in Texas, eventually ending up in Maryland. Along the way he pumped gas without paying for it. In Maryland a gas station attendant detained him and the police were forced to pick him up. This was my opportunity to get him into the hospital. The police called me because he was obviously mentally ill. I advised them to put him in the hospital. The sergeant told me that the police are not authorized to take anyone to the hospital in

Maryland. In actuality, making a responsible judgment, spending all day transporting him, with no arrest to count, is a bureaucratic non-starter. However, after a few hours of dealing with a psychotic person with manic depression, they decided to take him to the hospital even if it was not standard policy.

The lesson from this incident is that you can move the bureaucracy by putting an individual clerk into the position where doing nothing results in more work or thought than doing what needs to be done. With the police in Maryland I simply pointed this out. Often people will try to force this situation by complaining to a supervisor or threatening a lawsuit. I believe this approach is rarely effective.

A more positive approach is to find the individual bureaucrat who still thinks. This was exemplified when eventually my brother applied for social security disability. This assistance is difficult to obtain, takes many months and usually requires the assistance of a lawyer. In an obvious sense this is understandable. We do not want the government giving away our tax dollars without investigating the circumstances. The problem is that they don't really require an investigation but simply forms to be filled out. These lengthy and detailed forms require very little in the way of information that would help anyone understand the nature of a serious mental illness because they are designed for physical disabilities. Furthermore, people experiencing the disabilities associated with a manic or depressive episode cannot complete the paperwork in the first place. However, I had a long conversation with the social worker processing my brother's application. We discussed the history of his illness and the details of his disability. It was a conversation between two individuals, not an applicant with a representative of the state. The assistance was granted on the first application. But how many conversations like this are possible for any particular social worker? I had to call her; social workers do not attempt to contact the family. How much time is a social worker allotted for each case? Though the bureaucracy did not fail in this instance, it was only through unique circumstances that it succeeded.

Where should the power and responsibility for human problems be located? Raising children is largely left to parents, helping the poor has been subsumed by government, treating mental illness is a hodgepodge where many important decisions are constrained by bureaucracies. In all of these cases, an attempt to handle these human problems adequately requires intimate knowledge of the circumstances and character of the individuals involved. There is no question that the greatest knowledge and opportunity for therapy exists within the family. In a bygone era when most people lived in small communities people helped others as individuals. The village idiot or town drunk might not have received an income supplement, but they were known as individuals. It was not far-fetched to viewers of *Andy of Mayberry* that Otis the town drunk would be allowed to sleep off a bender in the jail.

I do not intend to romanticize the past; certainly there were many abuses of the mentally ill. Today intimate communities are few and far between. My brother often traveled thousands of miles in a psychotic state and so no community action would have been possible anyway. Furthermore, families are not always supportive. There are no easy answers. But it is only by allowing the lowest level of institutions in society such as families, churches, volunteer groups and civic organizations the freedom to make decisions, will there be any chance of treating manic depression fruitfully. This humane approach to human problems is very much in sync with the limited government and federalist principles of the U.S. Constitution and the Catholic principle of *subsidiarity.* Both traditions leave a sphere of freedom and responsibility to the lowest possible orders of society where bureaucracies and the clerk mentality are less prevalent.

It has been implicit in the arguments presented in this book that families will make decisions with the well-being of patients in mind. Of course this is not always the case for many reasons, as we have elucidated, and for the simple fact that families can include bad people. But I must emphasize that creating bureaucracies to overcome this shortcoming of the human condition has been an ultimate failure through history. It is the message here to move our society away from these so-called solutions.

chapter eight:

how does society deal with manic depression?

1. How does society deal with manic depression?

Stan: I have previously described manic depression, how it is treated and how it affects daily life. But this illness also has far-reaching implications for how patients function in the greater society. In each of the three phases of the illness (mania, hypomania and depression) there are distinct complications involved with interacting with various levels of society. I will describe these as they apply from my perspective in the following questions.

Ira: A key problem discussed in this book concerns the difficulty families have in understanding mental illness in general and manic depression in particular. This is even more of a problem for society at large. I would even contend that this is a problem for those directly charged by society to deal with manic depression, such as those in the judicial system. My experiences with many of these problems are recounted in the essays on my trip to Hawaii and bureaucracy located in Chapters 1 and 7, respectively. A more specific discussion of these issues is presented in this chapter.

2. What was your experience dealing with employers?

Stan: When I began my career as a physician I did not list manic depression as a condition that would interfere with my ability to practice medicine. My psychiatrist advised me that this was appropriate because I had suffered only one manic event that occurred before I began treating patients. Furthermore, I had been relatively stable and highly productive on medication (lithium) for three years. After completing medical school and receiving a Ph.D. in physiology, I began my medical internship. This is a demanding year of training, often requiring the intern to work overnight in the hospital. Once again,

I did extremely well, leading me to believe my illness was under control. However, a few months into the first year of my neurology residency I became manic, spending several months in and out of the hospital. Not one colleague attempted to contact me to demonstrate concern while I was recuperating. Even worse, while in the state mental hospital, I received a certified letter informing me of my dismissal. It is not that they were not a compassionate group. They did send a get-well card and flowers on behalf of the entire department only weeks earlier to the grandmother of a fellow resident who had fractured her hip. But I have learned not to expect any sympathy or aid due to my illness. Even my supervisor at another position, whose wife suffered from manic depression, had no understanding of how the illness affected my performance.

After my first residency I clearly noted my illness in all employment applications. I accepted positions where I thought I would receive the most support. I even asked them to set me up with a psychiatrist and expected a constructive communication between him and my supervisor. This never occurred, even during my psychiatry residency where my psychiatrist was also a member of the department.

As a consequence of this disease I have been fired five times. Four of these were secondary to having a manic episode. In the other instance, I did not go manic but suffered from depressions. This was my third neurology residency. The chairman who recruited me informed me that I could expect support from him and the faculty. Unfortunately, after accepting me for the position he notified me that he was leaving to study medical ethics at another institution. The irony was striking to me, like a hammer, but he was oblivious to it. Perhaps his subsequent studies have been beneficial to him. As a consequence there was nobody on the faculty to counterbalance those who felt I needed *special testing*. Thus, instead of support I faced discrimination and harassment from the first day. I strongly believe my depressions were exacerbated by the way the faculty treated me.

When I applied to be a physician in Mississippi, I reported that I had this illness on the application for my state medical license, which was approved. After starting my job I suffered from a relapse of mania. During my hospitalization a representative from the state medical board asked me to sign a document withdrawing my license, even though I was still manic. I followed my psychiatrist's advice to not comply. Several months later, when I had resumed my career in Texas, a letter arrived notifying me that there was to be a hearing regarding my license and that I was required to attend the hearing. Ira spoke to one of the board's lawyers and made it possible for me not to attend. He also sent a letter stating that I would not practice again in Mississippi without first appearing before the board. Supposedly this would mitigate the appearance of my name in the *National Practitioner Databank*, a published document that lists those physicians who have had negative actions taken against them-usually lawsuits. Despite our efforts to the contrary, the net effect was that my license was suspended (though as stated earlier I contractually could reapply) in Mississippi and my name did appear in the *Databank*. Thus, the net effect of my relations with employers in Mississippi and other places is that I have been treated as someone incompetent or criminal, not ill.

I believe that in being fired for an illness I was treated unfairly by my employers.

However, it is valid to question whether a person with manic depression can be dangerous on the job, especially in a medical setting, though one might also ask "Can you drive a car?" If one is stable and has a support system in place the answer is certainly "yes." It is true that if manic or depressed one's performance can be greatly affected. The loss of judgment and/or reality in both cases can induce harm. I believe that the individual with this disease will always require careful monitoring. This probably includes associates at the place of employment in addition to the family support structure.

Ira: In Chapter 6 I described my experience dealing with Stan's employers and my belief that only an employer who was also a friend would facilitate maintenance of a career. Eventually, I believe Stan will be able to resume working in a field related to his training. However, I think a necessary condition of his employment will be very flexible time commitments, be they daily, weekly or monthly. There are simply periods when Stan is disabled, by attempting to work through those periods in the past, he exacerbated his symptoms.

I believe the *Americans with Disabilities Act* is of no real use to those trying to work while suffering from manic depression. I suppose the intentions of those who passed it were good, as is the intention of most legislation; but it is fundamentally flawed, at least is terms of manic depression. The ADA proposes that persons are disabled if they are substantially limited in one or more of the major life activities. "Major life activities" means functions such as caring for oneself, performing manual tasks, walking, seeing, hearing, speaking, breathing, learning and *working* (my emphasis). Thus, if a baseball umpire should accidentally lose his eyesight, he would by definition of the ADA be disabled, not only because he cannot see but also because he cannot work. Therefore, by the ADA, he must be hired for the job that he cannot perform *precisely because he cannot perform it.* This is nonsense and counterproductive. In Stan's case he actually did go through periods when he could not perform his job. The difficulty is getting his employers to understand the nature of his illness. However, through the ADA, and lawsuits in general, we would much more likely become professional litigants than get Stan back in a productive work environment. The judicial system and the ADA are similar in that they are bureaucratic and thus are difficult for anyone to navigate successfully. This is especially the case for the mentally ill, as I described in Chapter 7. We discuss examples of particular experiences in our answers to a question to follow.

3. How does manic depression affect finances?

Stan: To say the least, bipolar disorder can have a devastating impact on personal and family finances. For the patient it is traumatic to lose financial independence. My family has initiated extreme measures to control my ability to inflict further financial damage upon myself. Because of my irresponsible purchases while manic, it has been necessary to limit my access to cash or credit. I do not have any major possessions. The car I drive, my apartment, bank accounts, all of my very limited assets are held in the name of my family for safekeeping.

I applied for and received social security disability several years after I became eligible. The delay was for two reasons. The first was that I was unaware that I was eligible for these benefits; no social worker or other professional in the hospital or out advised me. It was in a community support group that I received the information. My subsequent hesitation in applying was because I was too

ill to go through this long and relatively difficult process. There were several pages of
forms and the process takes months to complete, including an interview with a psychologist. Because of the difficulties involved in
obtaining these benefits, lawyers have practices devoted to aid applicants in this task. I
was apparently one of the fortunate few to
be approved on my first application and without legal assistance. However, the amount of
the disability compensation is not nearly adequate to sustain a decent living, especially
considering my medical expenses. Thus, I
applied for Medicaid for the poor. This arduous process involved much more paperwork.
In just the first year since this coverage has
started I have had five social workers handle
my case. When necessary, I have had to educate each one about the nature of my illness.

Returning to work would result in the loss
of benefits with both of these programs.
Should I have a relapse of the disease, the
entire application procedure would then have
to be repeated. Of course, this has a negative incentive to resuming employment.

Before I obtained Medicaid, I discovered

that no private insurance would offer me coverage for mental illness, and by and large, insurance companies will not underwrite patients with bipolar disorder for physical illnesses. Eventually I did find an agency that would give me some insurance for non-mental health coverage. Thankfully I did not need to use this coverage because this company declared bankruptcy shortly after I began my Medicaid coverage; thus I now question its legitimacy.

Ira: Manic depression is a disease that strikes at the financial health of patients and their families in several ways including loss of employment and thus loss of income, spending sprees on frivolous purchases that deplete savings, significant, continuing medical costs and, in Stan's case, discarding possessions while manic that subsequently had to be replaced. Furthermore, he also discarded his personal and family keepsakes that are irreplaceable.

Our family has cushioned the effects of this financial onslaught that amounts to tens of thousands of dollars. We assisted Stan in paying all of his debts resulting from spending sprees and medical treatment. We obviously wanted to help Stan in paying his debts, including maintaining a good credit rating for him. But we also felt a moral obligation as a family to pay off any debts incurred by any member of our family. However, I determined during his last major psychotic episode that paying those debts in effect subsidized the mania because wealth gives freedom that only resulted in trouble for Stan. Furthermore, with the moral obligation of paying off debts we expected some rights. For example, when we paid off credit-card bills we expected the credit-card companies to assist us if Stan were on a spending spree, at the minimum giving us information about his purchases. This assistance was given with extreme reluctance, if at all, even though I also had a power of attorney over Stan's finances. It was a typical pattern for businesses to take Stan's money while manic, often taking advantage of his flawed reasoning. When we attempted to intervene as his family, they told us Stan was an individual with rights that did not allow us legally to prevent him from wasting his money. In other words he was treated as an *atomized individual*, with no relations to family that were respected. Thus, we lost all our compulsion to pay Stan's debts to these businesses. This kind of behavior occurred with regard to rent on a condominium in Hawaii, a house in Mississippi and a car in

Texas for which he signed the sales papers as "God." A credit rating is an outmoded concept when an economy is awash in cheap money; with all of Stan's financial difficulties, he still receives pre-approved credit cards. Furthermore, it is dangerous for Stan to have such easy access to credit; for any other purchase, our family would rather have ownership, as I discuss below.

Currently Stan has no wealth of his own. All of the possessions he can use, including housing, transportation and food are owned, leased or purchased in some manner by a member of our family. All of his bank accounts are jointly held with a member of the family. In total, Stan has little to no financial independence. This is a situation we have come to very reluctantly after the years of experience we have described in this book. It is not a course of action I would suggest for all cases. It is an arrangement we might alter in the future. But I believe it is necessary for Stan at the moment, and it allows a family to have much greater control over the behavior of a manic depressive patient if he becomes psychotic. Families must consider such draconian measures for the protection of their loved ones who are ill.

4. What are the legal issues related to manic depression?

Stan: I have described the poor treatment I received from my employers in a previous answer. I have considered bringing a lawsuit to address my grievances. But I am not a contentious person by nature and until this illness developed, I had few problems in my life. When I was told my contract would not be renewed in my third neurology position I was encouraged by my family and my psychiatrist to hire a lawyer to allow me to complete my training. I knew I was more competent and definitely more concerned about the welfare of patients than at least some of the other residents. I did more than my share of work, was never absent and always punctual. I did not have a manic episode but my performance was not at my best at times because of mild depressions. I collected substantial documentation demonstrating my more-than-adequate performance. I provided this information to a lawyer who was recommended to me by my psychiatrist. I will refrain from a lawyer joke, but all he did was charge an exorbitant sum of money for sending a letter to the department. In my case, and I believe in more cases than not, lawsuits are a waste of time and money except for the lawyers.

I have also considered petitioning the government to assist me in dealing with employers. For example, does not the *Americans with Disabilities Act* apply in these cases? The act is vague, but in essence states that it is unlawful to discriminate against people who are handicapped physically as well as mentally. In my case, I find this law to be of little value. I am sure this is true for the vast majority of people with manic depression. The premise of the law in general is appealing, but I recognize it is appropriate to not hire someone with certain handicaps for specific jobs. This act does apply at times, or can be construed to apply, but it requires considerable effort to invoke its use.

The police are an important component of the legal system. I found the police reluctant to assist me even when I was disturbing to others. They seem to receive virtually no training regarding mental illness, and thus only relate to the illness as lay individuals. I was treated like a violent criminal in almost all instances. In one case in particular I was placed in overly tight handcuffs (which was common practice) that bruised and scratched my skin and shackles were placed around my ankles. Subsequently I developed a severe infection in one of my legs in a wound caused by the shackles. Furthermore, rough treatment by the police tended to exacerbate my troubled thoughts. I am thankful that in a few encounters with law enforcement they did get me to the hospital. In others, the police were satisfied if I would just follow their demand that I discontinue the specific behavior that warranted their call, and once I was hauled to jail.

Once in the hospital, all I wanted to do was get out if I was still manic. With the involuntary admissions the physician would always attempt to get me to sign a paper that this hospitalization would be voluntary. If not, a court hearing would supposedly ensue within a specified number of days. This did not always occur, and I do not know why, but I will let Ira discuss in detail how the judicial system manifested itself.

Ira: Over the years we have had dealings with the judicial system or police on many occasions. In most cases the relations have not been helpful; occasionally they have been detrimental and only rarely have they helped us help Stan. To repeat, this is due to the bureaucratic nature of these institutions and the fundamental misunderstanding of mental illness by society. Should Stan be classified as a normal citizen with civil rights, a criminal with civil rights or someone who is mentally ill with civil rights? And what are those rights in each instance? What rights and role does the family have with regard to legal issues? The people involved are usually not even cognizant of these difficult questions, and if so they are confused or reticent about how to answer them.

Consider first the critical, recurring problem of having a patient forcibly committed to a hospital. As I explain in the essay in Chapter 7, as bureaucratic institutions, the judicial system and police want to avoid anything to do with the mentally ill. Thus, to have Stan committed and remain hospitalized until his psychosis subsided was usually a difficult task. Virtually all of the professional medical *and* legal personnel I have encountered understood commitment to be based on whether or not Stan was *dangerous to himself or others.* Their understanding of this term was that Stan must be physically violent. As Stan has never been physically violent, this understanding has been a ready excuse for inaction, not that any particular excuse was needed for inaction. But we have described throughout this book that the dangers to Stan while manic are much more than simply physical violence. In fact, the concept of dangerous was even understood by the North Carolina legislature that passed the law on commitment as more than just physical violence. That law defines *dangerous to himself* as:

1. The individual has acted in such a way as to show:

   I. That he would be unable without care, supervision, and the continued assistance of others not otherwise available, to exercise self-control, judgement, and discretion in the conduct of his daily responsibilities and social relations, or to satisfy his need for nourishment, personal or medical care, shelter, or self-protection and safety; and

   II. That there is a reasonable probability of his suffering serious physical debilitation within the near future unless adequate treatment is given pursuant to this Chapter. A showing of behavior that is grossly inappropriate to the situation, or other evidence of severely impaired insight and judgement shall create a prima facie inference that the individual is unable to care for himself; or

2. The individual has attempted suicide of threatened suicide and that there is a reasonable probability of suicide unless adequate treatment is given pursuant to this Chapter; or

3. The individual has mutilated himself or attempted to mutilate himself and that there is a reasonable probability of serious self-mutilation unless adequate treatment is given pursuant to this Chapter. Previous episodes of dangerousness to self, when applicable, may be considered when determining reasonable probability of physical debilitation, suicide, or self-mutilation.

This law does reflect the full range of dangers to people suffering from manic depression, though I'm sorry that not every state has a comprehensive law. Even in North Carolina this definition is actually in another volume of the statutes than the law for commitment. However, I would have expected professionals to understand the complete meaning of the law. Unfortunately, this has not been the case, as described in the examples given below.

North Carolina Trial

In April of 1990 Stan was being treated in the Duke University Hospital. His recovery was not going well because he was not prevented from carrying out manic behavior. He refused all medication. He continuously called me and other members of our family. They were sick, scatological calls, totally out of his normal character. He was allowed to discard his wallet and contact lenses. In effect he was allowed to pursue the dangerous activities of Mr. Hyde. The confluence of circumstances of this poor care and the depletion of Stan's insurance coverage directed us toward transferring him to the state mental hospital in Butner, NC.

About a week after he was admitted to Butner, there was a hearing to determine if he was to remain there, which was required for all people admitted to the state hospital. I found out about it in the nick of time when I called the hospital to find out about Stan's condition. I had to rush to the hospital to attend, it being about an hour from Durham where I lived. It is important to note that I would not have been informed about this critical aspect of Stan's care if I had not called.

After arriving at the hospital I was directed to the foyer outside of the hearing room. It had a surreal atmosphere because of the many patients waiting for their hearings. Finally, after a couple of hours, Stan's hearing began. It was just like a regular court with a judge, district attorney, defendant (Stan), his lawyer (a public defender) and witnesses (his doctor and me). The district attorney first questioned the doctor who was a resident in his first court appearance. When asked if Stan were dangerous, he answered that he did not think so based on his observations. After trying to ask this question again a couple of more times, the district attorney said, "If he is not dangerous then this case is dismissed." I was flabbergasted. I literally jumped up and said I wanted to make a statement. I knew exactly what was happening; this psychiatrist did not understand the law. The district attorney obtained a recess and she, the doctor and myself had a consultation. I tried to explain to both of them that the doctor did not understand that the commitment law considered much more than just physical violence. Eventually I convinced the district attorney to show the doctor a copy of the law. Finally he understood and agreed to testify that Stan was dangerous in the legal sense. I also convinced the district attorney to allow me to speak. When the hearing resumed the doctor completed his testimony, now stating that Stan was dangerous to himself in the legal sense. Stan's lawyer cross-examined the psychiatrist to reinforce that he was not dangerous in the standard sense. I testified next. I do not recall the one question the district attorney asked me before I explained the history and implications of Stan's illness, including his throwing away his possessions, ruining his career because he did not believe in medicine and his contention that he was God. About 10 minutes later there really was no question in anyone's mind that Stan needed to be hospitalized. In sum, I said to the judge, "I am not testifying against Stan, I am testifying for him. He is ill and needs to be in the hospital." But we still had to go through with the rest of the hearing with Stan testifying last. In a twisted sense Stan was very logical. "Why did you throw your clothes away?" "They were old and I wanted new things." "Why did you quit medicine?" "The stress was too great and I wanted to do other things." Meanwhile I was thinking, please do not let him out, I can explain how these answers were based on his mania. Then he was asked, "Do you think you are God?" He answered "Yes, but I think a lot of people think like this." Finally in her closing statement, his lawyer stated that even if he thinks he is God he should not be held against his will. What could be more stupid and wrong? How could this public defender work to keep Stan from receiving the treatment he needed? I have found it is typical in these hearings that the professional participants, the "experts," have a poor understanding of mental illness in general and even less knowledge about the particulars of the case before them. Thankfully, the result of this surreal trial was that Stan "lost" and remained hospitalized.

Tennessee Trial

In Chapter 6, question 6 I described how I allowed Stan's last major psychotic episode to progress, expecting him soon to be hospitalized by the judicial system because he would become an irritant to society. My expectations were partially realized a couple of months after I decided on this approach.

I received a telephone call from a woman who had been a colleague of Stan's while in his residency position four years before at Vanderbilt University, located in Nashville, TN. Stan had driven to Nashville from San Antonio under the delusion that this woman was in love with him. He showed up on her doorstep in this condition. She knew of Stan's illness and somehow found my number to inform me of his presence in Nashville. She was now married, but her husband was traveling. She was frightened by the situation. I assured her that Stan had never been violent. But I also told her not to hesitate to call the police if she felt uncomfortable. In fact, I wanted Stan picked up by the police to be placed in a hospital. Thus it came to pass that Stan was arrested by the Nashville police.

I was contacted by a social worker at the jail informing me of Stan's incarceration. It was obvious that Stan was mentally ill, so he was not surprised when I explained the history of Stan's condition and that I wanted him admitted to a hospital. He explained to me that Stan would undergo a psychiatric evaluation to determine if he should stand trial or be sent to the mental hospital. To my great disappointment, the psychiatric evaluation consisted of only determining if Stan knew the name of the president and the year. The motivation for the negligence displayed by the psychiatrist making this evaluation was explained to me by the social worker. Two of the three public mental health hospitals had been closed in Davidson County. There was simply nowhere to put Stan but jail or back on the street.

It was approximately two weeks from the time Stan was picked up by the police until it was clear he would not be admitted to a hospital. I was in daily contact with the social worker over that time. We agreed that I had better come to Nashville to attend Stan's trial.

I flew to Nashville, found a room for the night, and first thing in the morning went to the jail downtown. I met with Stan. He was manic, and therefore uncooperative. A meeting of the judge, district attorney, social worker and myself ensued. It was my understanding that the charge against Stan would be dismissed if he went back to Texas with me and never returned to Tennessee. The authorities simply wanted to be rid of a problem. Of course Stan had to agree to these terms, which he did. Stan's compliance when confronted by the authority of the court is an example of how my strategy of attentive neglect described in Chapter 6 was intended to work. The approach failed in this case because the legal authority was not employed to make Stan well, but only to avoid dealing with a problem.

I described the trial in Butner as surreal. The day in court in Nashville was ridiculous. As I sat in the courtroom observing the criminal cases before Stan's, it became clear to me why truth and justice are such an elusive quarry when a bureaucratic system is the hunter. It seems nobody knew the facts, agreements or history of any of the cases. In contrast, Stan's court appearance was a model of efficiency and justice following our previous agreement.

Unfortunately, after this incident Stan did have a criminal record. First for just being arrested, in effect that is a conviction without a trial. And second, we found out years later that the record showed that he in fact pled guilty to stalking. I believe they simply screwed up the record, as I am positive the verbal agreement was to dismiss all the charges. Furthermore, the woman who made the charges was very sympathetic to Stan, sitting with me during the court proceedings.

The process of getting Stan released from jail and retrieving his impounded car and his luggage left at a motel was frustrating and exhausting. Frustrating because I had to follow the lead of Stan as Mr. Hyde. Exhausting because these errands took many hours to complete and required us to crisscross Nashville. The day consumed, in the midst of rush hour, we started back for Texas. I had to drive because Stan could not recover his wallet, including his driver's license. Was it stolen by the police as Stan contended? I don't know. In any case we drove all night to Texas. Stan did some driving after we left Tennessee. It was not until the next morning that we arrived in San Antonio. There was no occasion when Mr. Hyde disgusted me more than during this long drive through the night back to Texas.

From the examples I have recounted the picture of the legal-medical landscape comes into view. It is not a pretty picture. The medical community, and all other professionals, use a simplistic notion of the law to avoid difficult tasks related to treating manic depression. This also leads to a marginalization of the family in its efforts to have input into or perform these tasks themselves.

5. Is the government doing anything positive for the treatment of manic depression?

Ira: Certainly government should have a role in treating mental illness. I suggest that that role should be to empower the orders of society closest to the individual patient. Foremost must be the family, but the medical community is also hamstrung by government regulation or fear of lawsuits.

Funding of public mental hospitals is an important function for government because so many of the mentally ill are dangerous to themselves or others; therefore, these hospitals provide a service for all of society.

A more visible government effort has been the surgeon general's report on mental health. Its goal, greater awareness and understanding of mental illness among the general public, is much the same as the goal of this book. Unfortunately, the report lumps seemingly all problems of behavior as mental illness instead of considering character. Thus, the report is more a political ploy to expand an interest group than a fresh, positive approach to a difficult problem.

epilogue

The primary purpose of our writing this book was to provide therapy for Stan. As the body requires rehabilitation through physical exercise after an injury, we felt his brain needed mental exercise to recover from the trauma of extended mania and depression. This exercise has been arduous. He experienced a hypomanic episode while working on the book, perhaps due to the writing itself. Much more often he was unable to work due to the depressions which sapped his mental and physical energy. But overall he has made great progress in fighting his illness. He has not had a major manic episode in four years. His depressions have been less frequent and of less intensity during this period. I truly believe Stan will once again be able to use his many talents in a productive way, albeit with flexibility in his schedule so he can avoid periods of instability.

As difficult as this illness has been for Stan and our family, there are benefits that have come to us due to our trials. We are much closer than we would have been if Stan had not been ill. Because we are close I have had the privilege to observe my brother's great courage, the courage to deal with his illness and the courage to write about his ordeal. I am very proud to be Stan's brother.

We both hope this book will give the reader, either the patient or a loved one, the fundamental understanding and mindset to cope with this illness. The philosophy of the answers given is based on the common sense and stoicism gained by our experience and backed with the scientific, economic and social insight gained by our learning. However, it should be understood that these answers do not provide a complete response to this illness. To complete your understanding, to the limited extent that it is possible for anyone, this book should be supplemented by discussions with professionals and consultation with the other literature available. Even more apt, supplement the insights we have provided with your own, which will be gained through experience.

Ira Katz
January 2001